LOW-BUDGET GALVESTON DIET COOKBOOK FOR BEGINNERS

2000 Days Of Recipes: Delicious Galveston Flavors On A Budget! Discover Affordable Recipes Perfect For Health-Conscious Foodies, With A 30-Day Meal Plan

GRAYSON EMERSON

Table of Contents

CHAPTER ONE 4
   Introduction to the Galveston Diet on a Budget 4
   Understanding the Basics of the Galveston Diet 5
   Budget-Friendly Approaches to Healthy Eating 6
   Tips for Shopping Smart on a Budget 8

CHAPTER TWO 10
   Essential Pantry Staples 10
   Budget-Friendly Pantry Essentials 11
   Making the Most of Canned and Dry Goods 13
   DIY Seasoning Blends and Sauces 15

CHAPTER THREE 19
   Simple and Affordable Breakfasts 19

CHAPTER FOUR 25
   Budget-Friendly Lunches and Dinners 25

CHAPTER FIVE 32
   Thrifty Seafood Dishes 32

CHAPTER SIX 37
   Budget-Friendly Chicken Creations 37

CHAPTER SEVEN 43
   Economical Vegetable Delights 43

CHAPTER EIGHT 49
Affordable Snack Options 49
CHAPTER NINE 56
Budget-Friendly Desserts 56
CHAPTER TEN 61
Drinks and Beverages on a Budget 61
CHAPTER 11 66
A 31 MEAL PLAN 66
BONUS 74
SOME ESSENTIAL DIETS YOU SHOULD KNOW FOR HEALTHY LIVING 74
THE END 123

COPYRIGHT © 2023

All rights reserved. No part of this publication may be reproduced, distributed, or transmitted in any form or by any means, including photocopying, recording, or other electronic or mechanical methods, without the prior written permission of the publisher, except in the case of brief quotations embodied in critical reviews and certain other noncommercial uses permitted by copyright law.

CHAPTER ONE

Introduction to the Galveston Diet on a Budget

Embarking on a journey toward a healthier lifestyle often comes with a perceived barrier: cost. Many believe that eating healthy means spending more money, but the Galveston Diet challenges this notion by offering a practical approach to nutritious eating that won't break the bank. In this comprehensive guide, we'll delve into the fundamentals of the Galveston Diet and explore strategies for adopting it on a budget.

Understanding the Basics of the Galveston Diet

The Galveston Diet, developed by Dr. Mary Claire Haver, is a science-based eating plan designed specifically for women over 40 to optimize hormone balance and promote weight loss. It focuses on incorporating whole foods, healthy fats, lean proteins, and complex carbohydrates while minimizing processed foods, sugars, and artificial ingredients. The diet's emphasis on controlling insulin levels and reducing inflammation makes it conducive to overall health and well-being.

At the core of the Galveston Diet is the concept of intermittent fasting, which involves cycling between periods of eating and fasting. This approach not only aids in weight management but also enhances metabolic flexibility and improves cellular health. By abstaining from food for certain periods, the body can tap into stored fat for energy, leading to fat loss while preserving lean muscle mass.

In addition to intermittent fasting, the Galveston Diet advocates for mindful eating, emphasizing the importance of listening to hunger cues and eating slowly to promote digestion and satiety. By cultivating a mindful approach to eating, individuals can develop a healthier relationship with food and avoid overeating.

Another key component of the Galveston Diet is the inclusion of anti-inflammatory foods, such as leafy greens, berries, fatty fish, nuts, and seeds. These foods are rich in vitamins, minerals, and antioxidants, which help combat inflammation and support overall health. By prioritizing nutrient-dense foods, individuals can nourish their bodies and reduce the risk of chronic diseases.

While the Galveston Diet provides a framework for healthy eating, it's essential to personalize it based on individual needs and preferences. Some may thrive on a higher protein intake, while others may prefer a more plant-based approach. Experimenting with different foods and meal combinations can help individuals find what works best for them while still adhering to the principles of the Galveston Diet.

Budget-Friendly Approaches to Healthy Eating

Contrary to popular belief, eating healthy doesn't have to be expensive. With careful planning and strategic shopping, it's possible to follow the Galveston Diet without breaking the bank. Here are some budget-friendly approaches to consider:

1. **Meal Planning:** Planning meals in advance can help minimize food waste and ensure that ingredients are used efficiently. Start by creating a weekly meal plan based on budget-friendly recipes that align with the principles of the Galveston Diet. Look for affordable protein sources such as beans, lentils, eggs, and canned fish, and incorporate plenty of vegetables and whole grains to round out meals.

2. **Buy in Bulk:** Purchasing pantry staples like rice, beans, oats, and nuts in bulk can yield significant savings over time. Many grocery stores offer discounts for buying larger quantities, so take advantage of these deals to stock up on essentials. Consider joining a wholesale club or shopping at bulk food stores to access even greater savings on staple items.

3. **Shop Seasonally:** Buying fruits and vegetables that are in season is not only more economical but also ensures fresher, more flavorful produce. Seasonal produce tends to be abundant and therefore less expensive, making it a budget-friendly option for those following the Galveston Diet. Visit local farmers' markets or look for sales at supermarkets to score the best deals on seasonal produce.

4. **Utilize Frozen and Canned Foods:** Frozen fruits and vegetables are often more affordable than their fresh

counterparts and can be just as nutritious. Stock up on frozen berries, spinach, broccoli, and other staples to have on hand for quick and easy meals. Similarly, canned beans, tomatoes, and fish are budget-friendly pantry staples that can be used in a variety of dishes.

5. **Minimize Waste:** Reducing food waste is essential for maximizing your grocery budget. Use leftovers creatively by incorporating them into new meals or freezing them for later use. Additionally, make use of vegetable scraps to make homemade broth or compost them for gardening purposes. By being mindful of waste, you can stretch your food dollars further and minimize your environmental impact.

By implementing these budget-friendly approaches, individuals can enjoy the health benefits of the Galveston Diet without overspending. With a little planning and creativity, eating nutritious meals on a budget is entirely achievable.

Tips for Shopping Smart on a Budget

Navigating the grocery store can be overwhelming, especially when trying to stick to a budget. However, with some savvy shopping strategies, it's possible to make healthy choices without breaking the bank. Here are some tips for shopping smart on a budget:

1. **Make a List:** Before heading to the store, take inventory of what you already have on hand and make a list of the items

you need. Stick to your list while shopping to avoid impulse purchases and stay within your budget. Planning meals for the week can help determine which ingredients to include on your shopping list and prevent food waste.

2. **Compare Prices:** Don't assume that brand-name products are always the best value. Take the time to compare prices and consider purchasing store-brand or generic alternatives, which are often more budget-friendly. Look for sales, discounts, and coupons to further maximize your savings on essential items.

3. **Shop the Perimeter:** The perimeter of the grocery store is typically where fresh produce, meats, dairy, and other whole foods are located. Focus your shopping efforts on these areas, as they tend to offer the most nutrient-dense options. Limit your time in the center aisles, which are often filled with processed and packaged foods that may be more expensive and less nutritious.

4. **Buy in Bulk:** As mentioned earlier, buying certain items in bulk can result in significant cost savings over time. Look for bulk bins or larger package sizes for staples like grains, legumes, and spices. Just be sure to check the unit price to ensure you're getting the best value for your money.

5. **Stay Flexible:** While having a meal plan and shopping list is important, it's also essential to stay flexible and adaptable

while shopping. Keep an eye out for sales, markdowns, and clearance items that may not be on your list but offer excellent value. Be open to trying new foods and experimenting with different recipes based on what's available and affordable.

6. **Avoid Impulse Buys:** Grocery stores are designed to tempt you with enticing displays and promotions, making it easy to succumb to impulse purchases. To avoid overspending, stick to your list and resist the urge to buy items that aren't essential to your meal plan. If you're tempted by a particular item, take a moment to consider whether it's worth the extra cost or if there's a more budget-friendly alternative available.

By following these tips for shopping smart on a budget, individuals can make informed choices that support their health and financial goals. With a little planning and mindfulness, it's possible to eat well without breaking the bank, even when following the principles of the Galveston Diet.

CHAPTER TWO

Essential Pantry Staples

A well-stocked pantry is the cornerstone of a budget-friendly kitchen, providing the foundation for countless meals and snacks without the need for frequent trips to the grocery store. In this section, we'll explore the essential pantry staples that can help you create nutritious and satisfying meals while sticking to your budget.

Budget-Friendly Pantry Essentials

When it comes to stocking your pantry on a budget, prioritizing versatile and long-lasting ingredients is key. Here are some budget-friendly pantry essentials to consider:

1. **Grains:** Whole grains such as rice, quinoa, oats, and pasta are inexpensive staples that can serve as the foundation for a variety of meals. Opt for bulk packages or store-brand options to maximize savings.

2. **Legumes:** Beans, lentils, and chickpeas are affordable sources of protein, fiber, and essential nutrients. Dried varieties are typically more budget-friendly than canned, but canned options offer convenience and require less preparation.

3. **Canned Goods:** While fresh produce is ideal, canned goods can be a budget-friendly alternative, especially when certain

items are out of season. Stock up on canned tomatoes, beans, corn, and vegetables to have on hand for quick and easy meals.

4. **Oils and Vinegars:** Basic cooking oils like olive oil, vegetable oil, and coconut oil are pantry staples that can be used for sautéing, baking, and dressing. Similarly, vinegars such as balsamic, red wine, and apple cider can add flavor to salads, marinades, and sauces.

5. **Spices and Herbs:** Building a collection of dried spices and herbs allows you to add depth and complexity to your dishes without breaking the bank. Start with essentials like salt, pepper, garlic powder, onion powder, cumin, paprika, and oregano, then gradually expand your collection based on your cooking preferences.

6. **Broth and Stock:** Having broth or stock on hand is essential for adding depth and flavor to soups, stews, and sauces. While store-bought options are convenient, you can also make your own using vegetable scraps or leftover bones to save money.

7. **Nut Butters:** Peanut butter, almond butter, and other nut butters are nutritious and versatile pantry staples that can be used in both sweet and savory recipes. Look for natural or unsweetened varieties to avoid added sugars and preservatives.

8. **Canned Fish and Seafood:** Canned tuna, salmon, and sardines are budget-friendly sources of omega-3 fatty acids and protein. They can be used to make sandwiches, salads, pasta dishes, and more.

9. **Whole-Grain Flour:** Whether you're baking bread, muffins, or pancakes, having whole-grain flour on hand allows you to create healthier versions of your favorite treats. Look for whole wheat, oat, or almond flour for added nutritional benefits.

10. **Dried Fruit and Nuts:** Dried fruits like raisins, apricots, and cranberries are nutritious snacks that can also be used to add sweetness to oatmeal, baked goods, and salads. Similarly, nuts and seeds are packed with protein, healthy fats, and essential nutrients, making them an excellent pantry staple for snacking and cooking.

By stocking your pantry with these budget-friendly essentials, you'll be well-equipped to whip up delicious and nutritious meals without breaking the bank. With a little creativity and resourcefulness, you can make the most of these pantry staples to nourish yourself and your family on a budget.

Making the Most of Canned and Dry Goods

Canned and dry goods are pantry staples that offer convenience, versatility, and long shelf lives, making them essential components of a budget-friendly kitchen. Here are some tips for making the most of these pantry staples:

1. **Read Labels:** When purchasing canned goods, read labels carefully to avoid products that are high in sodium, sugar, or preservatives. Look for options with minimal added ingredients and opt for low-sodium or no-sugar-added varieties when possible.

2. **Rinse Canned Foods:** Canned beans, vegetables, and seafood often contain excess sodium and additives from the canning process. To reduce sodium content and improve flavor, rinse canned foods under cold water before using them in recipes.

3. **Use in Bulk:** Buying canned goods in bulk can yield significant savings over time, especially for items that you use frequently. Look for family-size or multipack options for staples like beans, tomatoes, and broth, and store extras in your pantry for future use.

4. **Stock Up During Sales:** Keep an eye out for sales and promotions on canned and dry goods at your local grocery store or online retailer. When items go on sale, consider stocking up on essentials to take advantage of lower prices and ensure that you always have pantry staples on hand.

5. **Repurpose Leftovers:** Leftover cooked grains, beans, and vegetables can be repurposed into new meals to minimize

waste and save money. Use leftover rice to make fried rice, toss cooked vegetables into soups or stir-fries, or mix beans into salads or grain bowls for added protein and fiber.

6. **Get Creative with Recipes:** Canned and dry goods are incredibly versatile and can be used in a wide range of recipes, from soups and stews to casseroles and salads. Experiment with different flavor combinations and ingredient pairings to create delicious and satisfying meals using pantry staples.

7. **Store Properly:** Properly storing canned and dry goods is essential for maintaining quality and freshness. Store canned foods in a cool, dry place away from direct sunlight, and use airtight containers to store dry goods like grains, beans, and flour to prevent moisture and pests from contaminating your pantry staples.

By following these tips, you can make the most of canned and dry goods in your pantry, saving money while still enjoying delicious and nutritious meals. With a little creativity and planning, you can transform these budget-friendly staples into satisfying dishes that nourish both body and soul.

DIY Seasoning Blends and Sauces

Creating your own seasoning blends and sauces at home is not only cost-effective but also allows you to control the quality and flavor of your ingredients. With a few basic pantry staples, you can whip up delicious and versatile seasonings and sauces to enhance your meals. Here are some DIY recipes to try:

1. **All-Purpose Seasoning Blend:**

- 1 tablespoon garlic powder
- 1 tablespoon onion powder
- 1 tablespoon dried oregano
- 1 tablespoon dried thyme
- 1 tablespoon paprika
- 1 teaspoon black pepper
- 1 teaspoon sea salt

Combine all ingredients in a small bowl and mix well. Store in an airtight container and use as a seasoning for meats, vegetables, soups, and more.

2. **Homemade BBQ Sauce:**

- 1 cup ketchup
- 1/4 cup apple cider vinegar
- 2 tablespoons honey or maple syrup
- 1 tablespoon Worcestershire sauce
- 1 teaspoon garlic powder

- 1 teaspoon onion powder
- 1/2 teaspoon smoked paprika
- 1/2 teaspoon chili powder
- Salt and pepper to taste

In a small saucepan, combine all ingredients over medium heat. Bring to a simmer and cook for 10-15 minutes, stirring occasionally, until the sauce has thickened. Adjust seasoning to taste and use as a marinade or dipping sauce for grilled meats, tofu, or vegetables.

3. **Italian Herb Dressing:**

- 1/4 cup extra-virgin olive oil
- 2 tablespoons red wine vinegar
- 1 clove garlic, minced
- 1 teaspoon dried oregano
- 1 teaspoon dried basil
- 1/2 teaspoon dried thyme
- 1/2 teaspoon dried rosemary
- Salt and pepper to taste

In a small bowl, whisk together olive oil, red wine vinegar, minced garlic, and dried herbs until well combined. Season with salt and pepper to taste. Drizzle over salads, grilled vegetables, or cooked pasta for a burst of flavor.

4. **Taco Seasoning Mix:**

- 1 tablespoon chili powder
- 1 teaspoon ground cumin
- 1 teaspoon smoked paprika
- 1/2 teaspoon garlic powder
- 1/2 teaspoon onion powder
- 1/2 teaspoon dried oregano
- 1/4 teaspoon cayenne pepper (optional)
- Salt and pepper to taste

Combine all ingredients in a small bowl and mix well. Use as a seasoning for tacos, burritos, quesadillas, or chili for a spicy and flavorful kick.

By making your own seasoning blends and sauces at home, you can save money on expensive store-bought versions while adding depth and complexity to your dishes. Experiment with different herbs, spices, and flavorings to create custom blends that suit your taste preferences and elevate your meals to new heights. With a well-stocked pantry and a little creativity, the possibilities are endless!

CHAPTER THREE

Simple and Affordable Breakfasts

Breakfast is often hailed as the most important meal of the day, providing the fuel and nutrients needed to kickstart your morning. However, busy schedules and tight budgets can make it challenging to prioritize a nutritious breakfast. In this section, we'll explore simple and affordable breakfast options that are both delicious and budget-friendly.

Budget-Friendly Overnight Oats

Overnight oats are a convenient and customizable breakfast option that can be prepared in advance and enjoyed on the go. With just a few basic ingredients, you can create delicious and nutritious overnight oats that won't break the bank. Here's how:

Ingredients:

- 1/2 cup rolled oats
- 1/2 cup milk (dairy or non-dairy)
- 1/4 cup yogurt (optional)
- 1 tablespoon chia seeds (optional)
- Sweetener of choice (honey, maple syrup, or stevia)
- Toppings such as fresh fruit, nuts, seeds, or nut butter

Instructions:

1. In a mason jar or container, combine rolled oats, milk, yogurt (if using), chia seeds (if using), and sweetener to taste. Stir well to combine.

2. Cover the jar or container and refrigerate overnight or for at least 4 hours to allow the oats to soften and absorb the liquid.

3. In the morning, give the oats a good stir and add your favorite toppings, such as fresh fruit, nuts, seeds, or nut butter.

4. Enjoy your delicious and nutritious overnight oats straight from the fridge or heat them up if desired.

Overnight oats can be customized to suit your taste preferences and dietary needs, making them a versatile and budget-friendly breakfast option. Experiment with different flavor combinations and toppings to keep things interesting and satisfying.

Quick and Easy Breakfast Egg Muffins

Breakfast egg muffins are a portable and protein-packed breakfast option that can be made ahead of time and enjoyed throughout the week. With just a few simple ingredients, you can whip up a batch of these tasty muffins in no time. Here's how:

Ingredients:

- 6 large eggs

- 1/4 cup milk (dairy or non-dairy)
- Salt and pepper to taste
- Fillings of choice (vegetables, cheese, cooked meat, etc.)

Instructions:

1. Preheat your oven to 350°F (175°C) and grease a muffin tin with cooking spray or olive oil.
2. In a large bowl, whisk together eggs, milk, salt, and pepper until well combined.
3. Divide the egg mixture evenly among the muffin cups, filling each cup about halfway full.
4. Add your desired fillings to each muffin cup, such as chopped vegetables, cheese, or cooked meat.
5. Bake the egg muffins in the preheated oven for 20-25 minutes, or until the eggs are set and the tops are lightly golden brown.
6. Allow the muffins to cool slightly before removing them from the muffin tin. Serve warm or let cool completely before storing in an airtight container in the refrigerator.

Breakfast egg muffins are incredibly versatile and can be customized with your favorite ingredients. They're perfect for meal prep and can be enjoyed hot or cold, making them a convenient and budget-friendly breakfast option for busy mornings.

Budget-Friendly Smoothie Recipes

Smoothies are a quick and easy way to pack in nutrients and energy in the morning, and they can be made on a budget with a few key ingredients. Here are some budget-friendly smoothie recipes to try:

1. **Green Banana Smoothie:**

   - 1 ripe banana
   - 1 cup spinach or kale
   - 1/2 cup Greek yogurt
   - 1/2 cup milk (dairy or non-dairy)
   - 1 tablespoon honey or maple syrup (optional)
   - Ice cubes (optional)

Instructions: Simply combine all ingredients in a blender and blend until smooth. Add more milk if needed to reach your desired consistency. Pour into glasses and enjoy immediately.

2. **Berry Oat Smoothie:**

   - 1/2 cup frozen mixed berries
   - 1/4 cup rolled oats

- 1/2 cup Greek yogurt
- 1/2 cup milk (dairy or non-dairy)
- 1 tablespoon honey or maple syrup (optional)

Instructions: Combine all ingredients in a blender and blend until smooth. Adjust sweetness to taste by adding more honey or maple syrup if desired. Pour into glasses and serve immediately.

3. **Peanut Butter Banana Smoothie:**

- 1 ripe banana
- 2 tablespoons peanut butter
- 1/2 cup Greek yogurt
- 1/2 cup milk (dairy or non-dairy)
- 1 tablespoon honey or maple syrup (optional)
- Ice cubes (optional)

Instructions: Combine all ingredients in a blender and blend until smooth. Add more milk if needed to reach your desired consistency. Pour into glasses and enjoy right away.

Smoothies are highly customizable, so feel free to experiment with different fruits, vegetables, and add-ins to create your own budget-friendly creations. By using affordable ingredients like frozen fruit, yogurt, milk, and oats, you can whip up nutritious and delicious smoothies without breaking the bank.

By incorporating these simple and affordable breakfast options into your morning routine, you can start your day off right without spending a fortune. Whether you prefer overnight oats, breakfast egg muffins, or budget-friendly smoothies, there's a delicious and nutritious breakfast option to suit every taste and budget.

CHAPTER FOUR

Budget-Friendly Lunches and Dinners

Creating satisfying and nutritious meals on a budget doesn't have to be complicated or time-consuming. With a few simple ingredients and some creative cooking techniques, you can whip up delicious lunches and dinners that won't break the bank. In this section, we'll explore budget-friendly recipes inspired by the Galveston Diet principles that are perfect for both lunch and dinner.

One-Pot Galveston Gumbo on a Budget

Gumbo is a classic Louisiana dish known for its rich flavor and hearty ingredients. This budget-friendly version of Galveston Gumbo captures the essence of the traditional recipe while using affordable ingredients and minimal prep time. Here's how to make it:

Ingredients:

- 1 tablespoon olive oil
- 1 onion, diced
- 2 cloves garlic, minced
- 1 bell pepper, diced
- 2 stalks celery, diced

- 1 pound smoked sausage, sliced
- 1 can diced tomatoes
- 4 cups chicken or vegetable broth
- 1 cup okra, sliced (fresh or frozen)
- 1 cup frozen shrimp, peeled and deveined
- 1 tablespoon Cajun seasoning
- Salt and pepper to taste
- Cooked rice for serving

Instructions:

1. In a large pot or Dutch oven, heat olive oil over medium heat. Add diced onion, garlic, bell pepper, and celery, and sauté until softened, about 5 minutes.
2. Add sliced smoked sausage to the pot and cook until lightly browned, about 5 minutes.
3. Stir in diced tomatoes, chicken or vegetable broth, sliced okra, and Cajun seasoning. Bring the mixture to a simmer and let it cook for 15-20 minutes, until the flavors have melded together and the okra is tender.
4. Add frozen shrimp to the pot and cook for an additional 5-7 minutes, until the shrimp are pink and cooked through.

5. Season the gumbo with salt and pepper to taste, and adjust the Cajun seasoning if desired.

6. Serve the Galveston Gumbo hot over cooked rice, garnished with chopped green onions or parsley if desired.

This budget-friendly Galveston Gumbo is a hearty and satisfying meal that's perfect for lunch or dinner. Packed with protein, fiber, and flavor, it's sure to become a family favorite without breaking the bank.

Budget-Friendly Veggie Stir-Fry

Stir-fries are a quick and versatile option for budget-friendly lunches and dinners, allowing you to use up leftover vegetables and proteins while packing in plenty of flavor and nutrition. This budget-friendly Veggie Stir-Fry is easy to customize based on what you have on hand and can be ready in under 30 minutes. Here's how to make it:

Ingredients:

- 2 tablespoons soy sauce
- 1 tablespoon rice vinegar
- 1 tablespoon honey or maple syrup
- 1 teaspoon sesame oil
- 1 tablespoon olive oil

- 2 cloves garlic, minced
- 1 tablespoon ginger, minced
- Assorted vegetables (such as bell peppers, broccoli, carrots, snap peas, and mushrooms), sliced or chopped
- Cooked protein of choice (such as tofu, chicken, shrimp, or tempeh)
- Cooked rice or noodles for serving

Instructions:

1. In a small bowl, whisk together soy sauce, rice vinegar, honey or maple syrup, and sesame oil to make the sauce. Set aside.
2. Heat olive oil in a large skillet or wok over medium-high heat. Add minced garlic and ginger, and sauté for 1-2 minutes until fragrant.
3. Add assorted vegetables to the skillet, starting with the ones that take longer to cook (such as carrots and broccoli) and adding quicker-cooking vegetables (such as bell peppers and snap peas) later.
4. Stir-fry the vegetables for 5-7 minutes, or until they are crisp-tender and slightly charred around the edges.

5. Add cooked protein of choice to the skillet and pour the sauce over the vegetables and protein. Stir well to coat everything evenly in the sauce.
6. Cook for an additional 2-3 minutes, until the sauce has thickened slightly and everything is heated through.
7. Serve the Veggie Stir-Fry hot over cooked rice or noodles, garnished with chopped green onions or sesame seeds if desired.

This budget-friendly Veggie Stir-Fry is a delicious and nutritious meal that's perfect for using up leftover vegetables and proteins. Feel free to customize it with your favorite ingredients and adjust the sauce to suit your taste preferences.

Rice and Beans Galveston Style

Rice and beans are a classic budget-friendly meal combination that's both nutritious and satisfying. This Galveston Style version adds extra flavor and protein to the dish, making it a delicious and filling option for lunch or dinner. Here's how to make it:

Ingredients:

- 1 tablespoon olive oil
- 1 onion, diced
- 2 cloves garlic, minced

- 1 bell pepper, diced
- 1 jalapeño pepper, seeded and diced (optional)
- 1 cup long-grain rice
- 2 cups chicken or vegetable broth
- 1 can black beans, drained and rinsed
- 1 teaspoon chili powder
- 1/2 teaspoon cumin
- Salt and pepper to taste
- Chopped cilantro for serving (optional)
- Lime wedges for serving (optional)

Instructions:

1. In a large skillet or saucepan, heat olive oil over medium heat. Add diced onion, minced garlic, diced bell pepper, and diced jalapeño pepper (if using), and sauté until softened, about 5 minutes.
2. Add long-grain rice to the skillet and cook, stirring frequently, for 2-3 minutes until lightly toasted.
3. Stir in chicken or vegetable broth, drained and rinsed black beans, chili powder, and cumin. Season with salt and pepper to taste.

4. Bring the mixture to a boil, then reduce the heat to low, cover, and simmer for 15-20 minutes, or until the rice is tender and the liquid has been absorbed.

5. Fluff the rice and beans with a fork, then serve hot, garnished with chopped cilantro and lime wedges if desired.

This budget-friendly Rice and Beans Galveston Style is a simple yet satisfying meal that's perfect for lunch or dinner. Packed with protein, fiber, and flavor, it's sure to become a go-to recipe for busy weeknights or meal prep sessions.

CHAPTER FIVE

Thrifty Seafood Dishes

Seafood dishes are often perceived as luxurious or expensive, but with some creativity and smart shopping, it's possible to enjoy delicious seafood meals on a budget. In this section, we'll explore thrifty seafood recipes that are both budget-friendly and bursting with flavor.

Budget-Friendly Shrimp Tacos

Shrimp tacos are a crowd-pleasing favorite that can easily be made on a budget by using simple ingredients and maximizing flavor. Here's how to whip up a batch of budget-friendly shrimp tacos:

Ingredients:

- 1 pound shrimp, peeled and deveined
- 1 tablespoon olive oil
- 1 teaspoon chili powder
- 1/2 teaspoon cumin
- 1/2 teaspoon paprika
- Salt and pepper to taste
- Corn or flour tortillas

- Toppings of choice (such as shredded cabbage, diced tomatoes, avocado slices, cilantro, lime wedges, and salsa)

Instructions:

1. In a large bowl, toss the peeled and deveined shrimp with olive oil, chili powder, cumin, paprika, salt, and pepper until evenly coated.

2. Heat a skillet or grill pan over medium-high heat. Add the seasoned shrimp to the pan and cook for 2-3 minutes per side, or until pink and cooked through.

3. Warm the tortillas in the skillet or microwave until soft and pliable.

4. Assemble the shrimp tacos by filling each tortilla with cooked shrimp and toppings of choice.

5. Serve the tacos hot, garnished with fresh cilantro and lime wedges for squeezing over the top.

These budget-friendly shrimp tacos are not only quick and easy to make but also packed with protein and flavor. Customize them with your favorite toppings and enjoy a delicious seafood meal without breaking the bank.

Baked Tilapia with Budget-Friendly Ingredients

Tilapia is a mild and versatile fish that lends itself well to budget-friendly meals. By baking tilapia with simple ingredients, you can create a delicious and nutritious dish that's perfect for a thrifty seafood dinner. Here's how:

Ingredients:

- 4 tilapia fillets
- 2 tablespoons olive oil
- 1 lemon, thinly sliced
- 2 cloves garlic, minced
- Salt and pepper to taste
- Fresh herbs for garnish (such as parsley or dill)

Instructions:

1. Preheat your oven to 400°F (200°C). Line a baking dish with parchment paper or foil for easy cleanup.

2. Place the tilapia fillets in the prepared baking dish and drizzle with olive oil. Season with minced garlic, salt, and pepper, then arrange lemon slices on top of each fillet.

3. Bake the tilapia in the preheated oven for 12-15 minutes, or until the fish is opaque and flakes easily with a fork.

4. Remove the tilapia from the oven and garnish with fresh herbs before serving.

This baked tilapia recipe is simple yet flavorful, allowing the natural taste of the fish to shine through. Pair it with steamed vegetables and rice for a complete and budget-friendly seafood dinner.

Tuna Salad Lettuce Wraps

Tuna salad lettuce wraps are a light and refreshing option for a budget-friendly seafood lunch or dinner. By using canned tuna and simple ingredients, you can create a satisfying meal that's both nutritious and delicious. Here's how:

Ingredients:

- 2 cans tuna, drained
- 1/4 cup mayonnaise or Greek yogurt
- 1 tablespoon Dijon mustard
- 1/4 cup diced celery
- 1/4 cup diced red onion
- 1 tablespoon chopped fresh dill or parsley
- Salt and pepper to taste
- Lettuce leaves for wrapping
- Sliced cucumber, avocado, or tomato for garnish (optional)

Instructions:

1. In a large bowl, combine drained tuna, mayonnaise or Greek yogurt, Dijon mustard, diced celery, diced red onion, and chopped fresh dill or parsley. Mix well to combine.

2. Season the tuna salad with salt and pepper to taste, adjusting the seasoning as needed.

3. Spoon the tuna salad onto lettuce leaves, dividing it evenly among the leaves.

4. Garnish the tuna salad lettuce wraps with sliced cucumber, avocado, or tomato if desired.

5. Roll up the lettuce leaves to form wraps and secure them with toothpicks if necessary.

6. Serve the tuna salad lettuce wraps immediately, or refrigerate them for later enjoyment.

These tuna salad lettuce wraps are a budget-friendly and satisfying option for lunch or dinner. Packed with protein and flavor, they're sure to become a staple in your meal rotation. Customize them with your favorite vegetables and enjoy a delicious seafood meal without breaking the bank.

CHAPTER SIX

Budget-Friendly Chicken Creations

Chicken is a versatile and budget-friendly protein that can be transformed into countless delicious dishes. In this section, we'll explore budget-friendly chicken recipes that are easy to make and bursting with flavor.

Budget-Friendly Baked Chicken Thighs

Baked chicken thighs are a simple and budget-friendly meal option that's perfect for busy weeknights. With just a few basic ingredients, you can create juicy and flavorful chicken thighs that the whole family will love. Here's how:

Ingredients:

- 4-6 chicken thighs, bone-in and skin-on
- 2 tablespoons olive oil
- 2 cloves garlic, minced
- 1 teaspoon paprika
- 1 teaspoon dried thyme
- 1 teaspoon dried rosemary
- Salt and pepper to taste

Instructions:

1. Preheat your oven to 400°F (200°C). Line a baking sheet with parchment paper or foil for easy cleanup.

2. In a small bowl, combine olive oil, minced garlic, paprika, dried thyme, dried rosemary, salt, and pepper. Mix well to create a flavorful marinade.

3. Place the chicken thighs on the prepared baking sheet and brush them generously with the marinade, making sure to coat both sides.

4. Bake the chicken thighs in the preheated oven for 25-30 minutes, or until the skin is crispy and golden brown and the internal temperature reaches 165°F (75°C).

5. Remove the chicken thighs from the oven and let them rest for a few minutes before serving.

These budget-friendly baked chicken thighs are delicious on their own or served with your favorite sides, such as roasted vegetables, mashed potatoes, or a fresh salad. They're perfect for meal prep and can be enjoyed hot or cold.

Budget-Friendly Chicken and Rice Casserole

Chicken and rice casserole is a comforting and satisfying dish that's perfect for feeding a crowd or meal prepping for the week ahead. This budget-friendly version of the classic recipe is made with simple ingredients and comes together quickly and easily. Here's how to make it:

Ingredients:

- 2 cups cooked chicken, shredded or diced
- 2 cups cooked rice
- 1 cup frozen mixed vegetables (such as peas, carrots, and corn)
- 1 can condensed cream of chicken soup
- 1/2 cup chicken broth
- 1/2 cup shredded cheddar cheese
- Salt and pepper to taste
- Optional toppings: crushed crackers or breadcrumbs for added crunch

Instructions:

1. Preheat your oven to 350°F (175°C). Grease a 9x13-inch baking dish with cooking spray or olive oil.
2. In a large bowl, combine cooked chicken, cooked rice, frozen mixed vegetables, condensed cream of chicken soup, chicken broth, shredded cheddar cheese, salt, and pepper. Mix well to combine.
3. Transfer the chicken and rice mixture to the prepared baking dish, spreading it out evenly.

4. If desired, sprinkle crushed crackers or breadcrumbs over the top of the casserole for added crunch and texture.

5. Bake the chicken and rice casserole in the preheated oven for 25-30 minutes, or until bubbly and golden brown on top.

6. Remove the casserole from the oven and let it cool for a few minutes before serving.

This budget-friendly chicken and rice casserole is a hearty and comforting meal that's perfect for feeding a hungry family. Feel free to customize it with your favorite vegetables and cheese for added flavor and nutrition.

Slow Cooker Chicken Chili

Chicken chili is a flavorful and satisfying dish that's perfect for chilly nights or game day gatherings. This budget-friendly version is made in the slow cooker, allowing the flavors to meld together while you go about your day. Here's how to make it:

Ingredients:

- 1 pound boneless, skinless chicken breasts or thighs
- 1 onion, diced
- 2 cloves garlic, minced
- 1 bell pepper, diced
- 1 can diced tomatoes

- 1 can black beans, drained and rinsed
- 1 can kidney beans, drained and rinsed
- 1 cup frozen corn
- 2 cups chicken broth
- 2 tablespoons chili powder
- 1 teaspoon cumin
- 1 teaspoon paprika
- Salt and pepper to taste
- Optional toppings: shredded cheese, sour cream, diced avocado, chopped cilantro, lime wedges

Instructions:

1. Place the chicken breasts or thighs in the bottom of a slow cooker. Add diced onion, minced garlic, diced bell pepper, diced tomatoes, black beans, kidney beans, frozen corn, chicken broth, chili powder, cumin, paprika, salt, and pepper.

2. Cover the slow cooker and cook on low for 6-8 hours or on high for 3-4 hours, until the chicken is tender and cooked through.

3. Remove the chicken from the slow cooker and shred it using two forks. Return the shredded chicken to the slow cooker and stir to combine.

4. Taste the chili and adjust the seasoning as needed, adding more salt, pepper, or chili powder if desired.

5. Serve the chicken chili hot, garnished with your favorite toppings such as shredded cheese, sour cream, diced avocado, chopped cilantro, and lime wedges.

This budget-friendly slow cooker chicken chili is packed with protein, fiber, and flavor, making it a hearty and satisfying meal for lunch or dinner. Serve it with cornbread, tortilla chips, or rice for a complete and delicious meal that won't break the bank.

CHAPTER SEVEN

Economical Vegetable Delights

Vegetables are not only nutritious but also versatile and budget-friendly. In this section, we'll explore economical vegetable recipes that are easy to make, packed with flavor, and gentle on the wallet.

Budget-Friendly Roasted Vegetables

Roasting vegetables is a simple and delicious way to bring out their natural sweetness and flavors. With just a few basic ingredients and minimal effort, you can create a colorful and nutritious side dish that complements any meal. Here's how to make budget-friendly roasted vegetables:

Ingredients:

- Assorted vegetables of your choice (such as carrots, potatoes, bell peppers, zucchini, broccoli, cauliflower, and Brussels sprouts)
- Olive oil
- Salt and pepper
- Optional seasonings (such as garlic powder, onion powder, paprika, or dried herbs)

Instructions:

1. Preheat your oven to 425°F (220°C). Line a baking sheet with parchment paper or foil for easy cleanup.

2. Wash and chop the vegetables into bite-sized pieces. Try to cut them into uniform sizes for even cooking.

3. Place the chopped vegetables in a large bowl and drizzle with olive oil, tossing to coat evenly. Season with salt, pepper, and any optional seasonings of your choice.

4. Spread the seasoned vegetables in a single layer on the prepared baking sheet, making sure they are not overcrowded.

5. Roast the vegetables in the preheated oven for 20-25 minutes, or until tender and caramelized, stirring halfway through cooking.

6. Remove the roasted vegetables from the oven and serve hot as a side dish or as part of a salad, grain bowl, or pasta dish.

These budget-friendly roasted vegetables are versatile and customizable, allowing you to use whatever vegetables you have on hand. They're perfect for meal prep and can be enjoyed hot or cold throughout the week.

Budget-Friendly Vegetable Soup

Vegetable soup is a comforting and nutritious meal that's perfect for using up leftover vegetables and pantry staples. This budget-friendly version of vegetable soup is hearty, flavorful, and easy to make. Here's how:

Ingredients:

- 1 tablespoon olive oil
- 1 onion, diced
- 2 cloves garlic, minced
- Assorted vegetables of your choice (such as carrots, celery, potatoes, tomatoes, green beans, peas, and corn), chopped
- 6 cups vegetable broth or chicken broth
- 1 can diced tomatoes
- 1 teaspoon dried herbs (such as thyme, oregano, or rosemary)
- Salt and pepper to taste

Instructions:

1. In a large pot or Dutch oven, heat olive oil over medium heat. Add diced onion and minced garlic, and sauté until softened and fragrant, about 5 minutes.
2. Add chopped vegetables to the pot and cook for an additional 5 minutes, stirring occasionally.

3. Pour vegetable broth and diced tomatoes into the pot, along with dried herbs, salt, and pepper. Bring the soup to a simmer.

4. Reduce the heat to low, cover the pot, and let the soup simmer for 20-25 minutes, or until the vegetables are tender.

5. Taste the soup and adjust the seasoning as needed, adding more salt and pepper if desired.

6. Serve the budget-friendly vegetable soup hot, garnished with fresh herbs if desired. Enjoy it as is or with a side of crusty bread or crackers for dipping.

This budget-friendly vegetable soup is a satisfying and nutritious meal that's perfect for lunch or dinner. Feel free to customize it with your favorite vegetables and herbs for added flavor and variety.

Stir-Fried Vegetables with Budget-Friendly Sauces

Stir-fried vegetables are a quick, easy, and budget-friendly way to enjoy the vibrant flavors and textures of fresh produce. By using simple sauces and seasonings, you can create delicious and nutritious stir-fries that are perfect for busy weeknights. Here's how:

Ingredients:

- Assorted vegetables of your choice (such as bell peppers, broccoli, carrots, snap peas, mushrooms, and onions), sliced or chopped

- Olive oil or sesame oil

- Garlic, minced

- Ginger, minced (optional)

- Soy sauce or tamari

- Rice vinegar

- Honey or maple syrup

- Cornstarch (optional, for thickening sauce)

- Optional toppings (such as sesame seeds, chopped green onions, or crushed red pepper flakes)

Instructions:

1. Heat olive oil or sesame oil in a large skillet or wok over medium-high heat. Add minced garlic and ginger (if using), and sauté for 1-2 minutes until fragrant.

2. Add sliced or chopped vegetables to the skillet or wok, starting with the ones that take longer to cook (such as carrots and broccoli) and adding quicker-cooking vegetables (such as bell peppers and snap peas) later.

3. Stir-fry the vegetables for 5-7 minutes, or until they are crisp-tender and slightly charred around the edges.

4. In a small bowl, whisk together soy sauce or tamari, rice vinegar, and honey or maple syrup to create a simple stir-fry sauce. You can also add cornstarch to thicken the sauce if desired.

5. Pour the sauce over the stir-fried vegetables and toss to coat evenly. Cook for an additional 1-2 minutes, until the sauce has thickened slightly and everything is heated through.

6. Remove the stir-fried vegetables from the heat and garnish with sesame seeds, chopped green onions, or crushed red pepper flakes if desired.

7. Serve the budget-friendly stir-fried vegetables hot over cooked rice or noodles, or enjoy them on their own as a light and healthy meal.

These budget-friendly stir-fried vegetables are versatile and customizable, allowing you to use whatever vegetables you have on hand. Experiment with different sauces and seasonings to create your own unique flavor combinations, and enjoy a delicious and nutritious meal that won't break the bank.

CHAPTER EIGHT

Affordable Snack Options

Snacking doesn't have to break the bank. With a little creativity and some smart shopping, you can enjoy delicious and satisfying snacks without spending a fortune. In this section, we'll explore budget-friendly snack options that are perfect for satisfying cravings between meals.

Budget-Friendly Trail Mix Recipes

Trail mix is a versatile and portable snack that's perfect for on-the-go munching. By making your own trail mix at home, you can customize the ingredients to suit your taste preferences and budget. Here are two budget-friendly trail mix recipes to try:

Recipe 1: Classic Nut and Fruit Trail Mix

Ingredients:

- 1 cup mixed nuts (such as almonds, peanuts, cashews, and walnuts)
- 1/2 cup dried fruit (such as raisins, cranberries, apricots, or banana chips)
- 1/4 cup chocolate chips or chunks (optional)
- 1/4 cup seeds (such as pumpkin seeds or sunflower seeds)

Instructions:

1. In a large bowl, combine mixed nuts, dried fruit, chocolate chips or chunks (if using), and seeds. Mix well to combine.

2. Transfer the trail mix to an airtight container or portion it out into individual snack bags for easy grab-and-go snacking.

3. Enjoy the classic nut and fruit trail mix as a satisfying and energy-boosting snack any time of day.

Recipe 2: Savory Spiced Trail Mix

Ingredients:

- 1 cup mixed nuts (such as almonds, cashews, and pecans)
- 1/2 cup pretzels or whole-grain crackers, broken into pieces
- 1/4 cup popcorn kernels, popped
- 1 tablespoon olive oil
- 1 teaspoon garlic powder
- 1 teaspoon onion powder
- 1/2 teaspoon smoked paprika
- Salt and pepper to taste

Instructions:

1. Preheat your oven to 300°F (150°C). Line a baking sheet with parchment paper.

2. In a large bowl, combine mixed nuts, pretzels or crackers, and popped popcorn.

3. Drizzle olive oil over the mixture and toss to coat evenly. Sprinkle with garlic powder, onion powder, smoked paprika, salt, and pepper, and toss again to coat.

4. Spread the seasoned trail mix in an even layer on the prepared baking sheet.

5. Bake the trail mix in the preheated oven for 15-20 minutes, stirring halfway through cooking, until the nuts are lightly toasted and the mixture is fragrant.

6. Remove the trail mix from the oven and let it cool completely before transferring it to an airtight container or portioning it out into individual snack bags.

These budget-friendly trail mix recipes are perfect for satisfying hunger cravings and providing a quick energy boost. Feel free to customize them with your favorite nuts, fruits, and seasonings for endless snacking possibilities.

Budget-Friendly Vegetable Sticks with Hummus

Vegetable sticks with hummus are a nutritious and satisfying snack that's perfect for munching between meals. By using budget-friendly vegetables and making your own hummus at home, you can create a delicious and affordable snack that's packed with flavor and nutrients. Here's how:

Ingredients:

- Assorted vegetables of your choice (such as carrots, cucumbers, bell peppers, celery, and cherry tomatoes), washed and cut into sticks or slices
- Homemade hummus (see recipe below) or store-bought hummus

Instructions:

1. Wash and cut the assorted vegetables into sticks or slices, making sure they are bite-sized and easy to dip.
2. Arrange the vegetable sticks on a platter or in a container for serving.
3. Serve the vegetable sticks with homemade hummus or store-bought hummus for dipping.
4. Enjoy the budget-friendly vegetable sticks with hummus as a nutritious and satisfying snack any time of day.

Homemade Hummus Recipe:

Ingredients:

- 1 can (15 ounces) chickpeas, drained and rinsed
- 2 tablespoons tahini (sesame seed paste)
- 2 tablespoons lemon juice

- 1 clove garlic, minced
- 2 tablespoons olive oil
- Salt and pepper to taste
- Water (as needed to achieve desired consistency)

Instructions:

1. In a food processor or blender, combine chickpeas, tahini, lemon juice, minced garlic, olive oil, salt, and pepper.
2. Blend until smooth, scraping down the sides of the bowl as needed. If the hummus is too thick, add water a tablespoon at a time until you reach your desired consistency.
3. Taste the hummus and adjust the seasoning as needed, adding more salt, pepper, or lemon juice if desired.
4. Transfer the homemade hummus to an airtight container and refrigerate for at least 30 minutes to allow the flavors to meld together.
5. Serve the homemade hummus with vegetable sticks for dipping, or use it as a spread for sandwiches, wraps, or crackers.

This budget-friendly snack option is not only delicious but also nutritious, providing a good source of fiber, vitamins, and minerals. Feel free to customize the vegetable sticks and hummus with your favorite flavors and ingredients for endless snacking enjoyment.

Budget-Friendly Fruit Salad

Fruit salad is a refreshing and nutritious snack that's perfect for satisfying sweet cravings. By using budget-friendly fruits and simple ingredients, you can create a delicious and affordable snack that's bursting with flavor and vitamins. Here's how to make a budget-friendly fruit salad:

Ingredients:

- Assorted fruits of your choice (such as apples, oranges, bananas, grapes, berries, melon, and pineapple), washed and chopped

- Optional add-ins (such as shredded coconut, chopped nuts, or a drizzle of honey or maple syrup)

- Optional garnishes (such as fresh mint leaves or a squeeze of lime juice)

Instructions:

1. Wash and chop the assorted fruits into bite-sized pieces, discarding any seeds or tough skins.

2. In a large bowl, combine the chopped fruits and any optional add-ins of your choice.

3. Toss the fruit salad gently to combine, making sure all the fruits are evenly distributed.

4. If desired, garnish the fruit salad with fresh mint leaves or a squeeze of lime juice for added flavor and freshness.

5. Serve the budget-friendly fruit salad immediately, or refrigerate it for later enjoyment.

This budget-friendly fruit salad is a delicious and nutritious snack option that's perfect for satisfying sweet cravings any time of day. Feel free to customize it with your favorite fruits and add-ins for endless snacking possibilities.

CHAPTER NINE

Budget-Friendly Desserts

Indulging in desserts doesn't have to break the bank. With a little creativity and some savvy shopping, you can enjoy delicious sweet treats without overspending. In this section, we'll explore budget-friendly dessert recipes that are easy to make and sure to satisfy your sweet tooth.

Budget-Friendly Banana Oat Cookies

Banana oat cookies are a healthy and budget-friendly alternative to traditional cookies. Made with simple ingredients and naturally sweetened with ripe bananas, these cookies are perfect for satisfying cravings without the guilt. Here's how to make them:

Ingredients:

- 2 ripe bananas, mashed
- 1 cup rolled oats
- 1/4 cup peanut butter or almond butter
- 1/4 cup chocolate chips or raisins (optional)
- 1/2 teaspoon cinnamon (optional)
- Pinch of salt

Instructions:

1. Preheat your oven to 350°F (175°C). Line a baking sheet with parchment paper.

2. In a large bowl, combine mashed bananas, rolled oats, peanut butter or almond butter, chocolate chips or raisins (if using), cinnamon (if using), and a pinch of salt. Mix well to combine.

3. Drop spoonfuls of the cookie dough onto the prepared baking sheet, leaving some space between each cookie.

4. Use a fork to flatten each cookie slightly.

5. Bake the cookies in the preheated oven for 12-15 minutes, or until lightly golden brown and set.

6. Remove the cookies from the oven and let them cool on the baking sheet for a few minutes before transferring them to a wire rack to cool completely.

These budget-friendly banana oat cookies are naturally sweet and satisfying, making them the perfect guilt-free dessert or snack. Enjoy them warm or at room temperature for a delicious treat that won't break the bank.

Budget-Friendly Fruit Sorbet

Fruit sorbet is a refreshing and light dessert that's perfect for hot summer days. By using budget-friendly fruits and simple ingredients, you can create a delicious and healthy treat that's sure to cool you down. Here's how to make it:

Ingredients:

- 4 cups frozen fruit of your choice (such as berries, mangoes, or peaches)
- 1/4 cup honey or maple syrup (optional, depending on the sweetness of the fruit)
- 2 tablespoons lemon juice
- 1/4 cup water (if needed to help blend)

Instructions:

1. Place the frozen fruit, honey or maple syrup (if using), and lemon juice in a food processor or blender.
2. Blend the ingredients until smooth and creamy, scraping down the sides of the bowl as needed. If the mixture is too thick to blend, add water a tablespoon at a time until you reach your desired consistency.
3. Taste the sorbet and adjust the sweetness if needed by adding more honey or maple syrup.
4. Transfer the sorbet to a shallow dish or container and freeze for at least 2-3 hours, or until firm.

5. Remove the sorbet from the freezer and let it sit at room temperature for a few minutes to soften slightly before scooping and serving.

This budget-friendly fruit sorbet is a refreshing and guilt-free dessert option that's perfect for satisfying cravings without breaking the bank. Experiment with different fruits and flavor combinations for endless variation.

Budget-Friendly Yogurt Parfaits

Yogurt parfaits are a simple and customizable dessert option that's perfect for using up leftover ingredients. By layering yogurt with budget-friendly toppings, you can create a delicious and satisfying treat that's sure to please. Here's how to make them:

Ingredients:

- Greek yogurt or your favorite yogurt variety
- Granola
- Fresh or frozen fruit (such as berries, bananas, or peaches)
- Honey or maple syrup (optional, for added sweetness)
- Nuts or seeds (such as almonds, walnuts, or pumpkin seeds)
- Optional toppings (such as shredded coconut, chocolate chips, or dried fruit)

Instructions:

1. Start by layering a spoonful of yogurt in the bottom of a glass or bowl.

2. Add a layer of granola on top of the yogurt, followed by a layer of fresh or frozen fruit.

3. Drizzle a little honey or maple syrup over the fruit if desired, for added sweetness.

4. Repeat the layers until you reach the top of the glass or bowl, finishing with a final layer of yogurt.

5. Sprinkle nuts or seeds on top of the parfait for added crunch and texture.

6. Garnish the yogurt parfait with optional toppings such as shredded coconut, chocolate chips, or dried fruit.

7. Serve the budget-friendly yogurt parfait immediately, or refrigerate it for later enjoyment.

These budget-friendly yogurt parfaits are versatile and customizable, allowing you to use whatever ingredients you have on hand. They're perfect for satisfying cravings while providing a good source of protein, calcium, and fiber. Enjoy them as a dessert or snack any time of day without breaking the bank.

CHAPTER TEN

Drinks and Beverages on a Budget

Staying hydrated doesn't have to be boring or expensive. With a little creativity and some budget-friendly ingredients, you can create refreshing and delicious drinks and beverages without breaking the bank. In this section, we'll explore three budget-friendly options that are perfect for quenching your thirst and satisfying your taste buds.

Budget-Friendly Infused Water Ideas

Infused water is a simple and refreshing way to add flavor to plain water without adding extra calories or sugar. By using budget-friendly fruits, vegetables, and herbs, you can create delicious infused water combinations that are perfect for staying hydrated throughout the day. Here are some budget-friendly infused water ideas to try:

1. **Cucumber and Mint Infused Water:** Thinly slice a cucumber and add it to a pitcher of water along with a handful of fresh mint leaves. Let the water sit in the refrigerator for a few hours to allow the flavors to infuse. Serve chilled over ice for a refreshing and hydrating drink.

2. **Lemon and Strawberry Infused Water:** Slice a lemon and hull and slice a handful of strawberries. Add the lemon slices and strawberries to a pitcher of water and let it sit in the

refrigerator for a few hours. The tangy lemon and sweet strawberries will infuse the water with flavor, creating a refreshing and thirst-quenching beverage.

3. **Watermelon and Basil Infused Water:** Cut fresh watermelon into cubes and tear a few basil leaves. Add the watermelon cubes and basil leaves to a pitcher of water and refrigerate for a few hours. The juicy watermelon and fragrant basil will infuse the water with a subtle sweetness and herbal aroma, making it a perfect summer drink.

4. **Citrus and Herb Infused Water:** Slice a combination of citrus fruits such as oranges, lemons, and limes, and add them to a pitcher of water along with a few sprigs of fresh herbs like rosemary or thyme. Let the water infuse in the refrigerator for several hours or overnight for a refreshing and aromatic drink.

These budget-friendly infused water ideas are not only delicious but also hydrating and refreshing, making them perfect for sipping throughout the day. Get creative with different fruit and herb combinations to find your favorite flavors.

Budget-Friendly Herbal Tea Blends

Herbal tea blends are a soothing and comforting beverage option that's perfect for relaxing and unwinding. By using budget-friendly herbs and spices, you can create delicious and flavorful tea blends that are perfect for any time of day. Here are some budget-friendly herbal tea blends to try:

1. **Chamomile and Lavender Tea:** Combine dried chamomile flowers and lavender buds in a tea infuser or tea bag. Steep the tea in hot water for 5-10 minutes, then strain and enjoy. The floral and calming flavors of chamomile and lavender make this tea perfect for bedtime or anytime you need to relax and unwind.

2. **Peppermint and Lemon Balm Tea:** Mix dried peppermint leaves and lemon balm leaves in a tea infuser or tea bag. Steep the tea in hot water for 5-7 minutes, then strain and enjoy. The refreshing and invigorating flavors of peppermint and lemon balm make this tea perfect for boosting energy and improving digestion.

3. **Ginger and Turmeric Tea:** Grate fresh ginger root and turmeric root into a tea infuser or tea bag. Steep the tea in hot water for 10-15 minutes, then strain and enjoy. The warming and spicy flavors of ginger and turmeric make this tea perfect for soothing sore throats and easing inflammation.

4. **Cinnamon and Cardamom Tea:** Crush cinnamon sticks and cardamom pods and add them to a tea infuser or tea bag. Steep the tea in hot water for 5-7 minutes, then strain and enjoy. The sweet and aromatic flavors of cinnamon and

cardamom make this tea perfect for satisfying sweet cravings without added sugar.

These budget-friendly herbal tea blends are easy to make and perfect for enjoying any time of day. Experiment with different herbs and spices to create your own unique flavor combinations.

Budget-Friendly Homemade Lemonade

Homemade lemonade is a classic and refreshing beverage option that's perfect for hot summer days. By using budget-friendly ingredients like lemons and sugar, you can create a delicious and thirst-quenching drink that's sure to please. Here's how to make it:

Ingredients:

- 1 cup freshly squeezed lemon juice (about 4-6 lemons)
- 1/2 cup granulated sugar
- 4 cups cold water
- Ice cubes
- Lemon slices and fresh mint leaves for garnish (optional)

Instructions:

1. In a small saucepan, combine granulated sugar with 1 cup of water. Heat over medium heat, stirring occasionally, until

the sugar has dissolved completely. Remove from heat and let the simple syrup cool to room temperature.

2. In a large pitcher, combine freshly squeezed lemon juice, cooled simple syrup, and cold water. Stir well to combine.

3. Taste the lemonade and adjust the sweetness by adding more sugar or water if needed.

4. Refrigerate the lemonade for at least 1 hour to chill before serving.

5. Serve the budget-friendly homemade lemonade over ice cubes, garnished with lemon slices and fresh mint leaves if desired.

This budget-friendly homemade lemonade is tangy, sweet, and refreshing, making it the perfect thirst-quenching beverage for any occasion. Feel free to customize it by adding other fruit juices or herbs for a unique twist.

CHAPTER 11

A 31 MEAL PLAN

Here's a 31-day meal plan to get you started:

Week 1:

Day 1:

- Breakfast: Scrambled eggs with spinach and mushrooms
- Lunch: Tuna salad lettuce wraps
- Dinner: Baked chicken thighs with roasted cauliflower

Day 2:

- Breakfast: Greek yogurt with berries and a sprinkle of chia seeds
- Lunch: Turkey and cheese roll-ups with cucumber slices
- Dinner: Zucchini noodles with marinara sauce and ground turkey

Day 3:

- Breakfast: Oatmeal with sliced banana and a drizzle of honey
- Lunch: Egg salad stuffed bell peppers
- Dinner: Baked salmon with steamed broccoli

Day 4:

- Breakfast: Smoothie with spinach, avocado, and almond milk
- Lunch: Chicken salad with mixed greens and cherry tomatoes
- Dinner: Beef stir-fry with bell peppers and broccoli, served over cauliflower rice

Day 5:

- Breakfast: Cottage cheese with pineapple chunks
- Lunch: Tuna avocado boats
- Dinner: Baked tilapia with roasted Brussels sprouts

Day 6:

- Breakfast: Whole grain toast with almond butter and sliced strawberries
- Lunch: Turkey and cheese lettuce wraps with mustard
- Dinner: Grilled chicken breast with sautéed spinach and garlic

Day 7:

- Breakfast: Scrambled eggs with diced bell peppers and onions
- Lunch: Cobb salad with grilled chicken, hard-boiled eggs, avocado, and bacon bits

- Dinner: Baked cod with lemon and herbs, served with a side of roasted asparagus

Day 8:

- Breakfast: Greek yogurt with sliced peaches and a sprinkle of granola
- Lunch: Turkey and cheese roll-ups with baby carrots and hummus
- Dinner: Baked chicken drumsticks with roasted sweet potatoes and green beans

Day 9:

- Breakfast: Overnight oats with almond milk, sliced banana, and a drizzle of maple syrup
- Lunch: Egg salad lettuce wraps with cherry tomatoes on the side
- Dinner: Baked cod with lemon butter sauce, served with quinoa and steamed broccoli

Day 10:

- Breakfast: Smoothie with spinach, frozen berries, Greek yogurt, and a splash of orange juice
- Lunch: Turkey and cheese stuffed bell peppers with salsa

- Dinner: Stir-fried tofu with mixed vegetables, served over brown rice

Day 11:

- Breakfast: Whole grain toast with avocado and a sprinkle of red pepper flakes
- Lunch: Tuna salad stuffed avocado halves
- Dinner: Baked pork chops with roasted Brussels sprouts and cauliflower

Day 12:

- Breakfast: Cottage cheese with sliced pear and a drizzle of honey
- Lunch: Chicken and vegetable skewers with tzatziki sauce
- Dinner: Baked tilapia with a squeeze of lemon, served with sautéed spinach

Day 13:

- Breakfast: Scrambled eggs with diced bell peppers, onions, and a sprinkle of shredded cheese
- Lunch: Cobb salad with grilled chicken, hard-boiled eggs, avocado, and ranch dressing
- Dinner: Beef and vegetable stir-fry with soy sauce, served over cauliflower rice

Day 14:

- Breakfast: Smoothie bowl with blended banana, spinach, almond milk, and topped with sliced almonds and shredded coconut
- Lunch: Turkey and cheese lettuce wraps with mustard and cucumber slices
- Dinner: Baked chicken thighs with roasted carrots and broccoli

Day 22:

- Breakfast: Greek yogurt with sliced strawberries and a drizzle of honey
- Lunch: Turkey and cheese roll-ups with a side of cherry tomatoes
- Dinner: Baked salmon with a squeeze of lemon, served with roasted asparagus and quinoa

Day 23:

- Breakfast: Oatmeal with mashed banana and a sprinkle of cinnamon
- Lunch: Egg salad lettuce wraps with cucumber slices
- Dinner: Grilled chicken breast with sautéed spinach and garlic, accompanied by roasted sweet potatoes

Day 24:

- Breakfast: Smoothie with spinach, frozen berries, Greek yogurt, and a splash of almond milk
- Lunch: Tuna salad stuffed tomatoes
- Dinner: Baked cod with a Mediterranean-inspired tomato and olive salsa, served with steamed broccoli

Day 25:

- Breakfast: Cottage cheese with diced pineapple and a sprinkle of chopped nuts
- Lunch: Turkey and cheese stuffed bell peppers with salsa
- Dinner: Beef stir-fry with bell peppers, broccoli, and snap peas, served over cauliflower rice

Day 26:

- Breakfast: Whole grain toast with mashed avocado and a poached egg
- Lunch: Chicken salad with mixed greens, cherry tomatoes, and balsamic vinaigrette
- Dinner: Baked pork chops with roasted Brussels sprouts and cauliflower

Day 27:

- Breakfast: Scrambled eggs with diced bell peppers and onions, topped with salsa

- Lunch: Cobb salad with grilled chicken, hard-boiled eggs, avocado, and ranch dressing

- Dinner: Grilled shrimp skewers with a squeeze of lemon, served with quinoa and sautéed spinach

Day 28:

- Breakfast: Smoothie bowl with blended banana, spinach, almond milk, and topped with sliced almonds and shredded coconut

- Lunch: Turkey and cheese lettuce wraps with mustard and cucumber slices

- Dinner: Baked chicken thighs with roasted carrots and broccoli

Day 29:

- Breakfast: Greek yogurt with sliced peaches and a sprinkle of granola

- Lunch: Tuna avocado boats

- Dinner: Baked tilapia with lemon butter sauce, served with quinoa and steamed green beans

Day 30:

- Breakfast: Overnight oats with almond milk, sliced banana, and a drizzle of maple syrup
- Lunch: Egg salad stuffed avocado halves
- Dinner: Beef and vegetable stir-fry with soy sauce, served over cauliflower rice

Day 31:

- Breakfast: Cottage cheese with sliced pear and a drizzle of honey
- Lunch: Chicken and vegetable skewers with tzatziki sauce
- Dinner: Baked salmon with a squeeze of lemon, served with roasted asparagus and cauliflower rice

BONUS

SOME ESSENTIAL DIETS YOU SHOULD KNOW FOR HEALTHY LIVING

Tofu Diet

Definition: The tofu diet involves incorporating tofu as a nutritious and versatile source of plant-based protein into meals. Tofu, also known as bean curd, is made from soybeans and is rich in protein, iron, calcium, and other nutrients. It is a staple in vegetarian and vegan diets due to its high protein content and ability to absorb flavors, making it a versatile ingredient in various cuisines.

Ingredients:

- **Tofu:** The star ingredient, rich in protein, iron, calcium, and other nutrients, serves as the foundation of this diet.

- **Vegetables:** Pair tofu with a variety of vegetables such as broccoli, bell peppers, spinach, or mushrooms for added flavor, texture, and nutrients.

- **Whole Grains:** Serve tofu alongside whole grains like brown rice, quinoa, or barley for added fiber and sustained energy.

- **Healthy Fats:** Incorporate sources of healthy fats such as olive oil, avocado, nuts, or seeds to enhance satiety and nutrient absorption.

- **Herbs and Spices:** Flavor tofu dishes with herbs, spices, and seasonings like garlic, ginger, soy sauce, or chili flakes to enhance taste and aroma.

Instructions:

1. **Stir-Fried Tofu:** Stir-fry cubed tofu with vegetables, garlic, ginger, and soy sauce for a quick and flavorful Asian-inspired dish that's perfect for busy weeknights.

2. **Tofu Scramble:** Crumble tofu and sauté with onions, peppers, spinach, and spices for a nutritious and satisfying alternative to scrambled eggs that's perfect for breakfast or brunch.

3. **Baked Tofu:** Marinate tofu slices in a mixture of soy sauce, maple syrup, and garlic, then bake until golden and crispy for a delicious and protein-packed main dish or salad topping.

4. **Tofu Bowl:** Build a tofu bowl with cooked tofu as the base, then top with vegetables, whole grains, avocado, and a drizzle of tahini or sriracha for a satisfying and customizable meal option.

5. **Tofu Soup:** Add cubed tofu to vegetable broth along with vegetables, noodles, and spices for a hearty and comforting soup that's perfect for cold weather or when you're feeling under the weather.

Tomatoes Diet

Definition: The tomatoes diet involves incorporating tomatoes as a nutritious and flavorful fruit into meals or snacks. Tomatoes are low in calories, rich in vitamins (such as vitamin C, vitamin K, and vitamin A), minerals (such as potassium and folate), and antioxidants (such as lycopene), making them a delicious and nutritious addition to any diet.

Ingredients:

- **Tomatoes:** The star ingredient, rich in vitamins, minerals, and antioxidants, serves as the foundation of this diet.

- **Other Vegetables:** Pair tomatoes with a variety of vegetables such as cucumbers, bell peppers, onions, or avocado for added flavor, texture, and nutrients.

- **Whole Grains:** Serve tomatoes alongside whole grains like whole wheat bread, brown rice, or quinoa for added fiber and sustained energy.

- **Healthy Fats:** Incorporate sources of healthy fats such as olive oil, avocado, nuts, or seeds to enhance satiety and nutrient absorption.

- **Herbs and Spices:** Flavor tomato dishes with herbs, spices, and seasonings like basil, oregano, garlic, or balsamic vinegar to enhance taste and aroma.

Instructions:

1. **Caprese Salad:** Layer sliced tomatoes with fresh mozzarella, basil leaves, and a drizzle of balsamic glaze for a simple and elegant salad that's perfect for summer.

2. **Tomato Soup:** Simmer tomatoes with onions, garlic, vegetable broth, and herbs until soft, then puree until smooth for a comforting and nutritious soup that's perfect for lunch or dinner.

3. **Tomato Bruschetta:** Top slices of toasted whole wheat bread with diced tomatoes, garlic, basil, and a drizzle of olive oil for a flavorful and satisfying appetizer or snack.

4. **Tomato Pasta:** Toss cooked pasta with diced tomatoes, garlic, spinach, and a touch of olive oil for a light and refreshing pasta dish that's perfect for summer.

5. **Stuffed Tomatoes:** Hollow out ripe tomatoes and fill with a mixture of cooked quinoa, vegetables, herbs, and cheese, then bake until tender for a delicious and nutritious vegetarian entree option.

Turkey Diet

Definition: The turkey diet involves incorporating turkey as a lean and protein-rich source into meals. Turkey is low in fat and calories while being high in protein, making it an excellent choice for those looking to increase their protein intake while managing their calorie intake. It also provides essential nutrients such as vitamins B6 and B12, niacin, zinc, and selenium.

Ingredients:

- **Turkey:** The star ingredient, rich in protein and low in fat, serves as the foundation of this diet.

- **Vegetables:** Pair turkey with a variety of vegetables such as spinach, kale, broccoli, or bell peppers for added nutrients, fiber, and flavor.

- **Whole Grains:** Serve turkey alongside whole grains like quinoa, brown rice, or whole wheat pasta for sustained energy and additional fiber.

- **Healthy Fats:** Incorporate sources of healthy fats such as olive oil, avocado, nuts, or seeds to enhance satiety and nutrient absorption.

- **Herbs and Spices:** Flavor turkey dishes with herbs, spices, and seasonings like garlic, rosemary, thyme, or paprika to enhance taste and aroma.

Instructions:

1. **Grilled Turkey Breast:** Grill turkey breast seasoned with herbs and spices until cooked through for a simple and delicious main dish that's perfect for summer barbecues.

2. **Turkey Stir-Fry:** Stir-fry sliced turkey breast with vegetables, garlic, ginger, and soy sauce for a quick and flavorful Asian-inspired dish that's perfect for busy weeknights.

3. **Turkey Salad:** Toss sliced turkey breast with mixed greens, avocado, walnuts, and a balsamic vinaigrette for a refreshing and nutrient-rich salad that's perfect for lunch or dinner.

4. **Turkey Wrap:** Wrap sliced turkey breast with lettuce, tomato, avocado, and hummus in a whole grain tortilla for a satisfying and portable meal option that's perfect for lunch or snacks.

5. **Turkey Chili:** Simmer ground turkey with tomatoes, beans, onions, and spices until flavors meld together for a hearty and nutritious chili that's perfect for cold weather or game days.

Walnuts Diet

Definition: The walnuts diet involves incorporating walnuts as a nutritious and heart-healthy nut into meals or snacks. Walnuts are rich in omega-3 fatty acids, antioxidants, vitamins (such as vitamin E), minerals (such as magnesium and copper), and fiber, making them a valuable addition to any diet.

Ingredients:

- **Walnuts:** The star ingredient, rich in omega-3 fatty acids, antioxidants, vitamins, minerals, and fiber, serves as the foundation of this diet.

- **Other Nuts and Seeds:** Pair walnuts with other nuts or seeds such as almonds, pecans, or chia seeds for added texture, flavor, and nutritional benefits.

- **Fruits:** Enjoy walnuts with fruits like apples, berries, or pears for a sweet and savory snack option that's rich in flavor and nutrients.

- **Whole Grains:** Serve walnuts alongside whole grains like oats, quinoa, or whole grain bread for added fiber and sustained energy.

- **Dairy or Dairy Alternatives:** Combine walnuts with Greek yogurt, almond milk, or cottage cheese for a creamy and nutritious breakfast or snack option.

Instructions:

1. **Raw Walnuts:** Enjoy raw walnuts on their own as a quick and convenient snack option that's packed with omega-3 fatty acids, antioxidants, and fiber.

2. **Walnut Trail Mix:** Combine walnuts with other nuts, seeds, dried fruits, and a sprinkle of dark chocolate chips for a flavorful and energizing trail mix that's perfect for hiking or snacking on the go.

3. **Walnut Salad:** Sprinkle chopped walnuts over mixed greens, sliced strawberries, goat cheese, and a balsamic vinaigrette for a refreshing and nutrient-rich salad that's perfect for lunch or dinner.

4. **Walnut Oatmeal:** Stir chopped walnuts into cooked oatmeal along with cinnamon, maple syrup, and a splash of almond milk for a hearty and satisfying breakfast option that's perfect for chilly mornings.

5. **Walnut Pesto:** Blend walnuts with basil, garlic, olive oil, Parmesan cheese, and lemon juice until smooth for a delicious and flavorful pesto sauce that's perfect for tossing with pasta, spreading on sandwiches, or topping grilled meats.

Watermelon Diet

Definition: The watermelon diet involves incorporating watermelon as a refreshing and hydrating fruit into meals or snacks. Watermelon is low in calories, high in water content, and packed with vitamins (such as vitamin C and vitamin A), minerals (such as potassium), and antioxidants (such as lycopene), making it a delicious and nutritious addition to any diet.

Ingredients:

- **Watermelon:** The star ingredient, rich in water, vitamins, minerals, and antioxidants, serves as the foundation of this diet.

- **Other Fruits:** Pair watermelon with other fruits such as berries, oranges, or kiwi for added flavor, sweetness, and variety.

- **Leafy Greens:** Toss watermelon chunks with mixed greens, feta cheese, mint, and a balsamic vinaigrette for a refreshing and nutrient-rich salad.

- **Mint:** Add fresh mint leaves to watermelon salads, smoothies, or agua frescas for a burst of freshness and flavor.

- **Citrus:** Squeeze lime or lemon juice over watermelon slices for a tangy and refreshing twist.

Instructions:

1. **Fresh Watermelon:** Enjoy chilled watermelon slices on their own as a refreshing and hydrating snack.

2. **Watermelon Smoothie:** Blend watermelon chunks with lime juice, mint leaves, and a splash of coconut water for a refreshing and hydrating smoothie that's perfect for hot days.

3. **Watermelon Salad:** Combine watermelon cubes with feta cheese, cucumber slices, red onion, and fresh mint leaves tossed in a lime vinaigrette for a refreshing and flavorful salad that's perfect for summer.

4. **Watermelon Gazpacho:** Blend watermelon chunks with tomatoes, cucumber, red bell pepper, red onion, garlic, and jalapeno until smooth, then chill for a refreshing and hydrating soup option that's perfect for warm weather.

5. **Watermelon Salsa:** Dice watermelon and combine with diced tomatoes, red onion, jalapeno, cilantro, lime juice, and a pinch of salt for a sweet and spicy salsa that's perfect for serving with grilled fish or chicken.

Zucchini Diet

Definition: The zucchini diet involves incorporating zucchini as a nutritious and versatile vegetable into meals. Zucchini is low in calories, rich in fiber, vitamins (such as vitamin C and vitamin K), minerals (such as potassium and manganese), and antioxidants, making it a valuable addition to any diet.

Ingredients:

- **Zucchini:** The star ingredient, rich in fiber, vitamins, minerals, and antioxidants, serves as the foundation of this diet.

- **Other Vegetables:** Pair zucchini with a variety of vegetables such as tomatoes, bell peppers, onions, or mushrooms for added flavor, texture, and nutrients.

- **Whole Grains:** Serve zucchini alongside whole grains like quinoa, brown rice, or whole wheat pasta for added fiber and sustained energy.

- **Proteins:** Pair zucchini with proteins like grilled chicken, tofu, chickpeas, or shrimp to create balanced and satisfying meals.

- **Herbs and Spices:** Flavor zucchini dishes with herbs, spices, and seasonings like garlic, basil, oregano, or red pepper flakes to enhance taste and aroma.

Instructions:

1. **Grilled Zucchini:** Slice zucchini lengthwise, brush with olive oil, sprinkle with salt and pepper, then grill until tender and slightly charred for a simple and delicious side dish that's perfect for summer barbecues.

2. **Zucchini Noodles:** Spiralize zucchini into noodles and toss with marinara sauce, garlic, and basil for a light and flavorful pasta alternative that's perfect for low-carb or gluten-free diets.

3. **Stuffed Zucchini:** Hollow out zucchini halves and fill with a mixture of cooked quinoa, vegetables, herbs, and cheese,

then bake until tender for a delicious and nutritious vegetarian entree option.

4. **Zucchini Stir-Fry:** Stir-fry sliced zucchini with other vegetables, tofu, or shrimp in a savory sauce made with soy sauce, garlic, ginger, and sesame oil for a quick and flavorful Asian-inspired dish that's perfect for weeknight dinners.

5. **Zucchini Fritters:** Grate zucchini and mix with eggs, breadcrumbs, Parmesan cheese, and herbs, then pan-fry until golden and crispy for a delicious and nutritious appetizer or snack option.

Almond Butter Diet

Definition: The almond butter diet involves incorporating almond butter as a nutritious and flavorful spread into meals or snacks. Almond butter is made from ground almonds and is rich in healthy fats, protein, fiber, vitamins (such as vitamin E and vitamin B2), minerals (such as magnesium and manganese), and antioxidants, making it a valuable addition to any diet.

Ingredients:

- **Almond Butter:** The star ingredient, rich in healthy fats, protein, fiber, vitamins, minerals, and antioxidants, serves as the foundation of this diet.

- **Fruits:** Pair almond butter with fruits such as apples, bananas, or berries for a sweet and satisfying snack option that's rich in flavor and nutrients.

- **Whole Grains:** Spread almond butter on whole grain toast, crackers, or rice cakes for a nutritious and energizing snack or breakfast option.

- **Smoothies:** Add a scoop of almond butter to smoothies along with fruits, leafy greens, nut milk, and a scoop of protein powder for a creamy and nutritious beverage that's perfect for breakfast or post-workout recovery.

- **Vegetables:** Dip vegetable sticks such as carrots, celery, or bell peppers into almond butter for a crunchy and satisfying snack option that's rich in fiber and nutrients.

Instructions:

1. **Almond Butter Toast:** Spread almond butter on whole grain toast and top with sliced bananas, a sprinkle of cinnamon, and a drizzle of honey for a delicious and nutritious breakfast option.

2. **Almond Butter Smoothie Bowl:** Blend almond butter with frozen bananas, spinach, almond milk, and a scoop of protein powder until smooth, then top with granola, berries, coconut flakes, and a drizzle of almond butter for a satisfying and Instagram-worthy breakfast or snack option.

3. **Almond Butter Energy Balls:** Mix almond butter with rolled oats, honey, and a touch of vanilla extract, then roll into balls and refrigerate until firm for a convenient and nutritious snack option that's perfect for on-the-go.

4. **Almond Butter Stir-Fry Sauce:** Whisk almond butter with soy sauce, garlic, ginger, and a splash of rice vinegar until smooth, then drizzle over stir-fried vegetables, tofu, or chicken for a creamy and flavorful sauce that's perfect for Asian-inspired dishes.

5. **Almond Butter Dressing:** Blend almond butter with lemon juice, olive oil, garlic, and herbs until smooth, then drizzle over salads or roasted vegetables for a creamy and flavorful dressing option that's rich in nutrients and flavor.

Almonds Diet

Definition: The almonds diet is a dietary approach that incorporates almonds as a primary component of meals or snacks. It often involves consuming almonds in various forms throughout the day to promote health and potentially aid in weight management.

Ingredients: Almonds are the central ingredient in the almonds diet. They are rich in healthy fats, protein, fiber, vitamins, and minerals. Additionally, the diet may include other foods such as fruits, vegetables, lean proteins, and whole grains to ensure a balanced nutrient intake.

Instructions:

1. **Incorporate Almonds Into Meals:** Include almonds in your breakfast, lunch, dinner, and snacks. For breakfast, add almonds to your cereal, yogurt, or oatmeal. For lunch and dinner, sprinkle almonds over salads or incorporate them into stir-fries and grain dishes.

2. **Snack on Almonds:** Keep a handful of almonds as a convenient and nutritious snack option. You can enjoy them on their own or pair them with fruits like apples or berries.

3. **Portion Control:** While almonds are nutritious, they are also calorie-dense. Practice portion control to avoid overconsumption, especially if your goal is weight management.

4. **Variety:** Experiment with different almond varieties such as raw, roasted, or flavored almonds to keep your meals interesting and flavorful.

5. **Stay Hydrated:** Drink plenty of water throughout the day, as almonds are naturally low in water content and hydration is essential for overall health and digestion.

Avocado Diet

Definition: The avocado diet emphasizes the inclusion of avocados as a significant component of meals. Avocados are known for their rich nutrient profile, including healthy fats, fiber, vitamins, and minerals.

Ingredients: Avocados are the main ingredient in the avocado diet. They can be used in various forms, including sliced, mashed, or blended into recipes. Other ingredients may include vegetables, lean proteins, whole grains, and healthy fats.

Instructions:

1. **Incorporate Avocados Into Meals:** Include avocados in your meals throughout the day. Add sliced avocado to sandwiches, wraps, and salads. Use mashed avocado as a spread on toast or as a topping for grilled proteins.

2. **Avocado Smoothies:** Blend avocado with fruits like bananas, berries, or spinach to create creamy and nutritious smoothies. You can also add protein powder or nut milk for an extra nutritional boost.

3. **Healthy Fats:** Avocados are rich in monounsaturated fats, which are beneficial for heart health. However, be mindful of portion sizes, as avocados are calorie-dense.

4. **Balanced Diet:** While avocados are nutritious, it's essential to maintain a balanced diet by including a variety of foods from all food groups.

5. **Enjoy in Moderation:** Avocados can be a healthy addition to your diet, but moderation is key. Monitor your portion sizes to avoid excessive calorie intake, especially if you're watching your weight.

Black Beans Diet

Definition: The black beans diet revolves around integrating black beans as a staple in meals to boost nutrition and promote overall health. Black beans are a type of legume rich in protein, fiber, vitamins, and minerals, making them a valuable addition to various dietary plans.

Ingredients:

- **Black Beans:** The primary ingredient, rich in protein and fiber, forms the cornerstone of this diet.

- **Vegetables:** Complement meals with a variety of vegetables for added nutrients and flavor.

- **Grains:** Incorporate whole grains like brown rice, quinoa, or whole wheat pasta for a balanced meal.

- **Lean Proteins:** Include lean proteins such as chicken, fish, or tofu to enhance the protein content and diversity of nutrients in your diet.

- **Herbs and Spices:** Flavor dishes with herbs, spices, and seasonings to enhance taste without relying on excessive salt or unhealthy additives.

Instructions:

1. **Include Black Beans in Meals:** Incorporate black beans into various meals, such as salads, soups, stews, burritos, tacos, or grain bowls.

2. **Diversify Your Recipes:** Experiment with different recipes and cuisines that feature black beans as a central ingredient. Explore Mexican, Cuban, or Southwestern-inspired dishes for variety.

3. **Combine with Complementary Foods:** Pair black beans with complementary foods to create balanced and satisfying meals. For example, combine black beans with rice for a complete protein source or add them to salads for extra fiber and protein.

4. **Watch Portion Sizes:** While black beans are nutritious, they are also calorie-dense. Be mindful of portion sizes, especially if you're watching your calorie intake or managing your weight.

5. **Prepare in Advance:** Cook a batch of black beans in advance and store them in the fridge or freezer for quick and convenient meal prep throughout the week.

Blueberries Diet

Definition: The blueberries diet emphasizes the consumption of blueberries as a primary source of antioxidants, vitamins, and fiber. Blueberries are renowned for their potential health benefits, including improved cognitive function, heart health, and management of blood sugar levels.

Ingredients:

- **Blueberries:** The star ingredient, packed with antioxidants and nutrients.

- **Other Fruits:** Incorporate a variety of fruits alongside blueberries to diversify nutrient intake and add natural sweetness to meals and snacks.

- **Dairy or Non-Dairy Products:** Pair blueberries with yogurt, milk, or dairy alternatives like almond milk for a nutritious breakfast or snack option.

- **Whole Grains:** Include whole grains such as oats, barley, or whole wheat toast to create balanced meals that provide sustained energy.

- **Nuts and Seeds:** Add nuts or seeds like almonds, walnuts, or chia seeds for additional nutrients and texture.

Instructions:

1. **Enjoy Blueberries Daily:** Aim to include blueberries in your daily diet by adding them to breakfasts, snacks, or desserts.

2. **Incorporate into Meals:** Add blueberries to oatmeal, yogurt bowls, smoothies, salads, or baked goods like muffins and pancakes.

3. **Mix with Other Fruits:** Combine blueberries with other fruits in salads, fruit bowls, or as toppings for yogurt or cereal to increase variety and nutrient intake.

4. **Experiment with Recipes:** Explore different recipes that feature blueberries as a central ingredient, such as blueberry chia pudding, blueberry smoothie bowls, or blueberry quinoa salad.

5. **Frozen Blueberries:** Keep frozen blueberries on hand to enjoy year-round and add them to recipes or snacks whenever fresh blueberries are not available.

Broccoli Diet

Definition: The broccoli diet focuses on incorporating broccoli as a prominent component of meals due to its high nutritional value. Broccoli is packed with vitamins, minerals, fiber, and antioxidants, making it a popular choice for those seeking to improve their overall health and well-being.

Ingredients:

- **Broccoli:** The main ingredient, rich in vitamin C, vitamin K, folate, and fiber.

- **Lean Proteins:** Include lean proteins such as chicken, fish, tofu, or legumes to create balanced meals.

- **Whole Grains:** Pair broccoli with whole grains like quinoa, brown rice, or whole wheat pasta for added fiber and nutrients.

- **Healthy Fats:** Incorporate sources of healthy fats like avocado, olive oil, nuts, or seeds to enhance nutrient absorption and satiety.

- **Herbs and Spices:** Flavor dishes with herbs, spices, and seasonings to enhance taste without relying on excessive salt or unhealthy additives.

Instructions:

1. **Include Broccoli in Meals:** Incorporate broccoli into various meals, such as stir-fries, salads, soups, casseroles, or as a side dish.

2. **Steam, Roast, or Saute:** Experiment with different cooking methods to prepare broccoli, such as steaming, roasting, or sautéing, to enhance flavor and texture.

3. **Pair with Protein:** Combine broccoli with lean proteins to create balanced and satisfying meals that provide a complete source of nutrients.

4. **Add Variety:** Explore different recipes and flavor combinations to keep meals interesting and enjoyable. Consider adding broccoli to pasta dishes, grain bowls, or frittatas.

5. **Meal Prep:** Prepare broccoli in advance and store it in the fridge for quick and convenient meal prep throughout the week. You can also freeze broccoli for longer-term storage.

Brussels Sprouts Diet

Definition: The Brussels sprouts diet centers around incorporating Brussels sprouts as a key ingredient in meals to boost nutrition and add variety to the diet. Brussels sprouts are a nutrient-dense vegetable rich in vitamins, minerals, fiber, and antioxidants, making them a valuable addition to any healthy eating plan.

Ingredients:

- **Brussels Sprouts:** The star ingredient, packed with vitamin K, vitamin C, folate, and fiber.

- **Other Vegetables:** Combine Brussels sprouts with other vegetables such as carrots, bell peppers, or cauliflower for added nutrients and flavor.

- **Proteins:** Pair Brussels sprouts with proteins like chicken, turkey, salmon, or tofu to create balanced and satisfying meals.

- **Whole Grains:** Serve Brussels sprouts alongside whole grains like quinoa, barley, or brown rice for added fiber and nutrients.

- **Healthy Fats:** Incorporate sources of healthy fats like olive oil, avocado, nuts, or seeds to enhance nutrient absorption and satiety.

Instructions:

1. **Prepare Brussels Sprouts:** Trim Brussels sprouts and cut them in half before cooking to ensure even cooking and enhanced flavor.

2. **Roast or Saute:** Roast Brussels sprouts in the oven with olive oil, garlic, and your favorite herbs and spices for a crispy and flavorful side dish. Alternatively, sauté Brussels sprouts with onions, garlic, and balsamic vinegar for a savory and delicious option.

3. **Pair with Protein:** Combine Brussels sprouts with lean proteins to create balanced meals that provide a complete source of nutrients. Try adding roasted Brussels sprouts to salads, grain bowls, or pasta dishes with grilled chicken or tofu.

4. **Experiment with Flavors:** Explore different flavor combinations by adding ingredients like bacon, maple syrup, Parmesan cheese, or dried cranberries to Brussels sprouts for added depth and complexity.

5. **Meal Prep:** Prepare a large batch of roasted Brussels sprouts and store them in the fridge for easy meal prep throughout the week. You can also freeze cooked Brussels sprouts for longer-term storage and convenience.

Chicken Diet

Definition: The chicken diet revolves around incorporating chicken as a primary source of lean protein in meals. Chicken is versatile, low in fat (especially if you remove the skin), and packed with essential nutrients like protein, vitamins, and minerals, making it a popular choice for those aiming to maintain or build muscle mass while keeping calorie intake in check.

Ingredients:

- **Chicken:** The main ingredient, providing a lean source of protein.

- **Vegetables:** Pair chicken with a variety of vegetables to increase fiber intake and add essential vitamins and minerals to meals.

- **Whole Grains:** Serve chicken alongside whole grains like brown rice, quinoa, or whole wheat pasta for sustained energy and additional fiber.

- **Healthy Fats:** Incorporate sources of healthy fats such as avocado, olive oil, nuts, or seeds to enhance satiety and nutrient absorption.

- **Herbs and Spices:** Flavor chicken dishes with herbs, spices, and seasonings to add depth and complexity to the flavors without relying on excessive salt or unhealthy additives.

Instructions:

1. **Choose Lean Cuts:** Opt for lean cuts of chicken such as chicken breast or skinless chicken thighs to minimize saturated fat intake.

2. **Grill, Bake, or Broil:** Cook chicken using healthy cooking methods like grilling, baking, or broiling to minimize added fats and calories.

3. **Add Flavor:** Marinate chicken with herbs, spices, citrus juice, or yogurt-based marinades to infuse flavor and tenderize the meat before cooking.

4. **Pair with Vegetables:** Serve chicken with a generous portion of vegetables to create balanced and nutritious meals. Try roasted vegetables, stir-fried veggies, or a colorful salad.

5. **Meal Prep:** Prepare batches of grilled or baked chicken in advance and portion them out for easy meal prep throughout the week. You can also freeze cooked chicken for longer-term storage and convenience.

Chia Seeds Diet

Definition: The chia seeds diet incorporates chia seeds as a nutritional powerhouse into meals to boost fiber, protein, omega-3 fatty acids, and various micronutrients. Chia seeds are versatile and can be easily added to a wide range of dishes, making them a convenient addition to any diet.

Ingredients:

- **Chia Seeds:** The star ingredient, rich in fiber, protein, omega-3 fatty acids, and antioxidants.

- **Liquid:** Mix chia seeds with liquids such as water, milk (dairy or plant-based), yogurt, or fruit juice to create chia seed pudding or beverages.

- **Fruits:** Pair chia seeds with fruits like berries, bananas, or mangoes for added flavor, sweetness, and additional nutrients.

- **Nuts and Seeds:** Combine chia seeds with nuts or seeds such as almonds, walnuts, or pumpkin seeds for added texture and nutritional variety.

- **Sweeteners (Optional):** Add natural sweeteners like honey, maple syrup, or agave nectar if desired, but keep in mind the added sugar content.

Instructions:

1. **Chia Seed Pudding:** Mix chia seeds with your choice of liquid (e.g., almond milk) and sweetener (if desired), then let it sit in the fridge overnight to thicken into a pudding-like consistency. Serve with fresh fruit or nuts for added flavor and texture.

2. **Smoothies:** Blend chia seeds into smoothies along with fruits, leafy greens, protein powder, and your choice of liquid for a nutritious and filling beverage.

3. **Salads and Yogurt:** Sprinkle chia seeds over salads or yogurt bowls to add crunch, fiber, and omega-3 fatty acids.

4. **Baking:** Incorporate chia seeds into baked goods like muffins, bread, or energy bars for added nutrition and texture. Chia seeds can be used as an egg substitute in vegan baking recipes.

5. **Hydration:** Mix chia seeds into water or flavored beverages to create a hydrating chia seed drink. The seeds absorb liquid and develop a gel-like consistency, providing sustained hydration and a boost of nutrients.

Cottage Cheese Diet

Definition: The cottage cheese diet involves incorporating cottage cheese as a central component of meals or snacks. Cottage cheese is a low-fat dairy product rich in protein, calcium, and other essential nutrients. It's often used by individuals aiming to increase protein intake, promote muscle growth, and support weight loss or management.

Ingredients:

- **Cottage Cheese:** The primary ingredient, rich in protein and calcium, serves as the foundation of this diet.

- **Fruits:** Pair cottage cheese with fruits like berries, peaches, or pineapple for added flavor, natural sweetness, and additional vitamins and minerals.

- **Vegetables:** Combine cottage cheese with vegetables such as cucumbers, tomatoes, or bell peppers for a savory twist and increased fiber content.

- **Whole Grains:** Serve cottage cheese alongside whole grains like whole wheat crackers or bread for added fiber and sustained energy.

- **Herbs and Spices:** Flavor cottage cheese with herbs, spices, or seasonings like black pepper, dill, or chives to enhance taste without relying on excessive salt or unhealthy additives.

Instructions:

1. **Simple Snack:** Enjoy cottage cheese on its own as a quick and convenient snack option.

2. **Fruit Parfait:** Layer cottage cheese with your favorite fruits and a drizzle of honey or maple syrup to create a delicious and nutritious parfait.

3. **Salad Topping:** Use cottage cheese as a topping for salads instead of traditional dressings. It adds creaminess and protein to your salad while keeping the calorie count lower.

4. **Smoothies:** Blend cottage cheese into smoothies along with fruits, leafy greens, and your choice of liquid for a protein-rich beverage.

5. **Stuffed Vegetables:** Use cottage cheese as a filling for stuffed vegetables like bell peppers or tomatoes, along with herbs, spices, and other veggies for added flavor and nutrition.

Cucumbers Diet

Definition: The cucumbers diet emphasizes the consumption of cucumbers as a primary vegetable in meals or snacks. Cucumbers are low in calories, refreshing, and hydrating, making them an excellent choice for those looking to increase vegetable intake, support hydration, and promote weight loss or management.

Ingredients:

- **Cucumbers:** The star ingredient, low in calories and high in water content, serves as the foundation of this diet.

- **Dressing or Dip:** Pair cucumbers with healthy dressings or dips such as hummus, Greek yogurt-based dips, or vinaigrettes for added flavor and creaminess.

- **Proteins:** Combine cucumbers with protein sources like grilled chicken, tofu, or chickpeas to create balanced and satisfying meals.

- **Whole Grains:** Serve cucumbers alongside whole grains like quinoa, brown rice, or farro for added fiber and sustained energy.

- **Herbs and Spices:** Flavor cucumbers with herbs, spices, or seasonings like mint, dill, or lemon zest to enhance taste and aroma.

Instructions:

1. **Simple Snack:** Enjoy sliced cucumbers on their own as a refreshing and hydrating snack option.

2. **Salads:** Incorporate cucumbers into salads alongside other vegetables, greens, proteins, and grains for a nutritious and filling meal.

3. **Cucumber Cups:** Use cucumber slices or hollowed-out cucumber halves as cups to hold fillings like tuna salad,

chicken salad, or hummus for a fun and creative appetizer or snack.

4. **Pickles:** Make homemade pickles by soaking cucumber slices in a mixture of vinegar, water, salt, and spices for a tangy and crunchy snack.

5. **Cucumber Water:** Infuse water with cucumber slices and fresh herbs like mint or basil for a refreshing and hydrating beverage option.

Egg Diet

Definition: The egg diet involves incorporating eggs as a primary source of protein in meals. Eggs are nutrient-dense, rich in high-quality protein, vitamins, minerals, and healthy fats. This diet is often used for weight loss, muscle building, or as part of a balanced eating plan.

Ingredients:

- **Eggs:** The main ingredient, providing high-quality protein, essential vitamins (such as vitamin B12 and vitamin D), and minerals (such as iron and selenium).

- **Vegetables:** Pair eggs with a variety of vegetables like spinach, bell peppers, tomatoes, or mushrooms for added fiber, vitamins, and minerals.

- **Whole Grains:** Serve eggs alongside whole grains such as whole wheat toast, quinoa, or oatmeal for sustained energy and additional fiber.

- **Healthy Fats:** Incorporate sources of healthy fats like avocado, olive oil, nuts, or seeds to enhance satiety and nutrient absorption.

- **Herbs and Spices:** Flavor egg dishes with herbs, spices, and seasonings like black pepper, paprika, or fresh herbs to add depth and complexity to the flavors.

Instructions:

1. **Basic Preparation:** Enjoy eggs cooked in various ways, such as boiled, poached, scrambled, fried (using minimal oil), or baked, depending on personal preference.

2. **Omelets:** Make omelets by whisking eggs with vegetables, cheese, and herbs, then cooking them in a skillet until set. Customize omelets with your favorite fillings for a nutritious and satisfying meal.

3. **Frittatas:** Bake eggs with vegetables and cheese in a frittata for a simple and versatile dish that can be enjoyed for breakfast, lunch, or dinner.

4. **Egg Salad:** Prepare egg salad by mixing chopped hard-boiled eggs with Greek yogurt, mustard, celery, and spices. Serve

on whole grain bread or lettuce wraps for a protein-rich meal.

5. **Meal Prep:** Boil a batch of eggs in advance and store them in the fridge for easy meal prep throughout the week. Hard-boiled eggs make a convenient and portable snack or addition to salads and sandwiches.

Fish Diet

Definition: The fish diet involves incorporating various types of fish into meals to reap the health benefits associated with consuming seafood. Fish is rich in high-quality protein, omega-3 fatty acids, vitamins, and minerals, making it a valuable component of a healthy eating plan.

Ingredients:

- **Fish:** Choose a variety of fish species such as salmon, tuna, trout, mackerel, sardines, or cod to enjoy a diverse range of flavors and nutrients.

- **Vegetables:** Pair fish with a variety of vegetables like leafy greens, broccoli, asparagus, or zucchini for added fiber, vitamins, and minerals.

- **Whole Grains:** Serve fish alongside whole grains like brown rice, quinoa, or barley for sustained energy and additional fiber.

- **Healthy Fats:** Fish itself is a source of healthy fats, particularly omega-3 fatty acids, which are beneficial for heart health. Supplement with additional sources of healthy fats like avocado, olive oil, nuts, or seeds as desired.

- **Herbs and Spices:** Flavor fish dishes with herbs, spices, and seasonings like garlic, lemon, dill, or thyme to enhance taste and aroma.

Instructions:

1. **Grilled Fish:** Grill fish fillets or whole fish with a drizzle of olive oil and a sprinkle of herbs and spices for a simple and flavorful dish.

2. **Baked Fish:** Bake fish fillets with lemon slices, garlic, and herbs for a light and healthy meal that's easy to prepare.

3. **Fish Tacos:** Prepare fish tacos by grilling or baking fish, then serving it in corn or whole wheat tortillas with cabbage slaw, avocado, salsa, and a squeeze of lime for a delicious and nutritious meal.

4. **Fish Curry:** Make fish curry by simmering fish with coconut milk, tomatoes, onions, and spices for a flavorful and comforting dish that pairs well with rice or naan.

5. **Canned Fish:** Incorporate canned fish like tuna or salmon into salads, sandwiches, or pasta dishes for a convenient and

budget-friendly protein option that's rich in omega-3 fatty acids.

Flaxseeds Diet

Definition: The flaxseeds diet involves incorporating flaxseeds as a nutritional powerhouse into meals to boost fiber, protein, omega-3 fatty acids, and various micronutrients. Flaxseeds are versatile and can be easily added to a wide range of dishes, making them a convenient addition to any diet.

Ingredients:

- **Flaxseeds:** The star ingredient, rich in fiber, protein, omega-3 fatty acids, and antioxidants.

- **Liquid:** Mix ground flaxseeds with liquids such as water, milk (dairy or plant-based), yogurt, or fruit juice to create a flaxseed gel or add them directly into smoothies, oatmeal, or yogurt for added nutrition.

- **Fruits:** Pair flaxseeds with fruits like berries, bananas, or apples for added flavor, sweetness, and additional nutrients.

- **Nuts and Seeds:** Combine flaxseeds with nuts or seeds such as almonds, walnuts, or pumpkin seeds for added texture and nutritional variety.

- **Sweeteners (Optional):** Add natural sweeteners like honey, maple syrup, or agave nectar if desired, but keep in mind the added sugar content.

Instructions:

1. **Flaxseed Gel:** Mix ground flaxseeds with water to create a flaxseed gel, which can be used as an egg substitute in baking recipes or as a thickening agent in sauces and dressings.

2. **Smoothies:** Blend ground flaxseeds into smoothies along with fruits, leafy greens, protein powder, and your choice of liquid for a nutritious and filling beverage rich in omega-3 fatty acids and fiber.

3. **Oatmeal:** Stir ground flaxseeds into cooked oatmeal along with fruits, nuts, and spices for a hearty and nutritious breakfast option.

4. **Baking:** Incorporate ground flaxseeds into baked goods like muffins, bread, or energy bars for added nutrition and texture. Flaxseeds can be used as an egg substitute in vegan baking recipes.

5. **Yogurt Topping:** Sprinkle ground flaxseeds over Greek yogurt along with fruits, nuts, and a drizzle of honey or maple syrup for a nutritious and satisfying snack or breakfast option.

Greek Yogurt Diet

Definition: The Greek yogurt diet involves incorporating Greek yogurt as a central component of meals or snacks due to its high protein content, probiotics, and versatility. Greek yogurt is a strained yogurt that has a thicker consistency and higher protein content compared to regular yogurt, making it a popular choice for those seeking to increase protein intake and support gut health.

Ingredients:

- **Greek Yogurt:** The main ingredient, rich in protein, probiotics, calcium, and other essential nutrients.

- **Fruits:** Pair Greek yogurt with fruits like berries, peaches, or mangoes for added flavor, natural sweetness, and additional vitamins and minerals.

- **Nuts and Seeds:** Combine Greek yogurt with nuts or seeds such as almonds, walnuts, or chia seeds for added texture, healthy fats, and nutritional variety.

- **Honey or Maple Syrup (Optional):** Add natural sweeteners like honey or maple syrup to Greek yogurt if desired, but keep in mind the added sugar content.

- **Whole Grains:** Serve Greek yogurt alongside whole grains like granola, oats, or whole grain cereal for added fiber and sustained energy.

Instructions:

1. **Simple Snack:** Enjoy Greek yogurt on its own as a quick and convenient snack option.

2. **Parfait:** Layer Greek yogurt with your favorite fruits, nuts, seeds, and a drizzle of honey or maple syrup to create a delicious and nutritious parfait.

3. **Smoothies:** Blend Greek yogurt into smoothies along with fruits, leafy greens, protein powder, and your choice of liquid for a protein-rich beverage that's creamy and satisfying.

4. **Salad Dressing:** Use Greek yogurt as a base for salad dressings by mixing it with lemon juice, herbs, spices, and a touch of olive oil for a creamy and tangy dressing option.

5. **Dips:** Combine Greek yogurt with herbs, spices, and seasonings to create savory dips for vegetables, crackers, or pita bread. Greek yogurt-based dips are a healthier alternative to sour cream-based dips and are rich in protein and probiotics.

Green Beans Diet

Definition: The green beans diet involves incorporating green beans as a primary vegetable in meals to boost nutrition and add variety to the diet. Green beans are low in calories, rich in fiber, vitamins (such as vitamin C, vitamin K, and folate), and minerals (such as manganese and potassium), making them a valuable addition to any healthy eating plan.

Ingredients:

- **Green Beans:** The star ingredient, low in calories and high in fiber, vitamins, and minerals, serves as the foundation of this diet.

- **Proteins:** Pair green beans with proteins like grilled chicken, tofu, fish, or lean beef to create balanced and satisfying meals.

- **Whole Grains:** Serve green beans alongside whole grains like quinoa, brown rice, or whole wheat pasta for added fiber and sustained energy.

- **Healthy Fats:** Incorporate sources of healthy fats such as olive oil, avocado, nuts, or seeds to enhance nutrient absorption and satiety.

- **Herbs and Spices:** Flavor green beans with herbs, spices, and seasonings like garlic, lemon, dill, or thyme to enhance taste and aroma.

Instructions:

1. **Steamed Green Beans:** Steam green beans until tender-crisp and season with a sprinkle of salt, pepper, and a drizzle of olive oil for a simple and nutritious side dish.

2. **Green Bean Salad:** Blanch green beans in boiling water, then toss with cherry tomatoes, red onion, feta cheese, and a balsamic vinaigrette for a refreshing and colorful salad.

3. **Stir-Fry:** Stir-fry green beans with garlic, ginger, soy sauce, and your choice of protein for a quick and flavorful Asian-inspired dish.

4. **Roasted Green Beans:** Roast green beans in the oven with olive oil, garlic, and Parmesan cheese for a crispy and savory side dish that pairs well with grilled meats or fish.

5. **Green Bean Casserole:** Prepare a classic green bean casserole with green beans, cream of mushroom soup, and crispy fried onions for a comforting and nostalgic dish that's perfect for holidays or special occasions.

Kale Diet

Definition: The kale diet emphasizes the consumption of kale as a nutrient-rich leafy green vegetable in meals or snacks. Kale is packed with vitamins, minerals, fiber, and antioxidants, making it one of the healthiest foods you can eat.

Ingredients:

- **Kale:** The star ingredient, rich in vitamins (such as vitamin A, vitamin K, and vitamin C), minerals (such as calcium and potassium), fiber, and antioxidants.

- **Fruits:** Pair kale with fruits like berries, apples, or oranges for added flavor, sweetness, and additional nutrients.

- **Nuts and Seeds:** Combine kale with nuts or seeds such as almonds, walnuts, or sunflower seeds for added texture, healthy fats, and nutritional variety.

- **Whole Grains:** Serve kale alongside whole grains like quinoa, farro, or barley for added fiber and sustained energy.

- **Proteins:** Pair kale with proteins like grilled chicken, salmon, tofu, or chickpeas to create balanced and satisfying meals.

Instructions:

1. **Kale Salad:** Massage kale with lemon juice and olive oil to soften the leaves, then toss with your favorite toppings such as avocado, nuts, seeds, and a flavorful dressing for a nutritious and satisfying salad.

2. **Kale Smoothie:** Blend kale into smoothies along with fruits, Greek yogurt, nut milk, and a scoop of protein powder for a green smoothie that's packed with vitamins, minerals, and fiber.

3. **Kale Chips:** Toss kale leaves with olive oil, salt, and your choice of seasonings, then bake in the oven until crispy for a healthy and crunchy snack alternative to potato chips.

4. **Kale Soup:** Simmer kale with vegetables, beans, and broth to create a hearty and nutritious soup that's perfect for cold weather or when you're feeling under the weather.

5. **Stir-Fry:** Stir-fry kale with garlic, ginger, soy sauce, and your choice of protein for a quick and flavorful Asian-inspired dish that's perfect for busy weeknights.

Kiwi Diet

Definition: The kiwi diet involves incorporating kiwi fruit as a primary source of vitamins, minerals, and antioxidants into meals or snacks. Kiwi is renowned for its high vitamin C content, as well as its fiber, potassium, and vitamin K, making it a nutritious addition to any diet.

Ingredients:

- **Kiwi:** The star ingredient, rich in vitamin C, fiber, potassium, and antioxidants, serves as the foundation of this diet.

- **Other Fruits:** Pair kiwi with other fruits such as berries, oranges, or pineapple for added flavor, sweetness, and variety.

- **Greek Yogurt:** Combine kiwi with Greek yogurt for a creamy and nutritious breakfast or snack option that's rich in protein and probiotics.

- **Nuts and Seeds:** Sprinkle chopped kiwi over nuts or seeds like almonds, walnuts, or chia seeds for added texture, healthy fats, and nutritional variety.

- **Whole Grains:** Serve kiwi alongside whole grains like oatmeal, quinoa, or whole grain toast for added fiber and sustained energy.

Instructions:

1. **Kiwi Salad:** Combine sliced kiwi with mixed greens, avocado, nuts, seeds, and a balsamic vinaigrette for a refreshing and nutrient-rich salad.

2. **Kiwi Smoothie:** Blend kiwi into smoothies along with other fruits, leafy greens, Greek yogurt, nut milk, and a scoop of protein powder for a green smoothie that's packed with vitamins, minerals, and protein.

3. **Kiwi Salsa:** Dice kiwi and combine with chopped tomatoes, onions, cilantro, jalapeno, lime juice, and a pinch of salt for a flavorful and refreshing salsa that pairs well with grilled fish or chicken.

4. **Kiwi Parfait:** Layer chopped kiwi with Greek yogurt, granola, and a drizzle of honey or maple syrup for a nutritious and satisfying parfait that's perfect for breakfast or dessert.

5. **Kiwi Sorbet:** Blend frozen kiwi with a splash of orange juice and a touch of honey or agave syrup until smooth, then freeze until firm for a refreshing and healthy dessert option.

Lentils Diet

Definition: The lentils diet involves incorporating lentils as a versatile and nutritious legume into meals to boost protein, fiber, vitamins, and minerals intake. Lentils are an excellent source of plant-based protein, making them a valuable addition to vegetarian and vegan diets.

Ingredients:

- **Lentils:** The star ingredient, rich in protein, fiber, vitamins (such as folate and vitamin B6), and minerals (such as iron and magnesium), serves as the foundation of this diet.

- **Vegetables:** Pair lentils with a variety of vegetables such as carrots, onions, tomatoes, spinach, or bell peppers for added flavor, texture, and nutrients.

- **Whole Grains:** Serve lentils alongside whole grains like brown rice, quinoa, or whole wheat couscous for added fiber and sustained energy.

- **Herbs and Spices:** Flavor lentil dishes with herbs, spices, and seasonings like garlic, cumin, coriander, or smoked paprika to enhance taste and aroma.

- **Healthy Fats:** Incorporate sources of healthy fats such as olive oil, avocado, nuts, or seeds to enhance satiety and nutrient absorption.

Instructions:

1. **Lentil Soup:** Simmer lentils with vegetables, broth, and seasonings to create a hearty and nutritious soup that's perfect for cold weather or when you're feeling under the weather.

2. **Lentil Salad:** Toss cooked lentils with mixed greens, chopped vegetables, herbs, nuts, seeds, and a vinaigrette for a refreshing and satisfying salad that's packed with plant-based protein and fiber.

3. **Lentil Curry:** Cook lentils with coconut milk, tomatoes, onions, garlic, ginger, and curry spices for a flavorful and comforting curry dish that pairs well with rice or naan.

4. **Lentil Stew:** Combine lentils with root vegetables, tomatoes, broth, and herbs in a slow cooker or Instant Pot for a hearty and nourishing stew that's easy to prepare and perfect for meal prep.

5. **Lentil Tacos:** Fill taco shells or tortillas with seasoned lentils, lettuce, tomatoes, avocado, salsa, and a squeeze of lime for a tasty and nutritious meatless taco option that's suitable for vegetarians and vegans.

Mango Diet

Definition: The mango diet emphasizes the incorporation of mangoes as a primary source of vitamins, minerals, and antioxidants into meals or snacks. Mangoes are renowned for their high vitamin C content, as well as their fiber, vitamin A, and potassium, making them a delicious and nutritious addition to any diet.

Ingredients:

- **Mango:** The star ingredient, rich in vitamin C, vitamin A, fiber, and antioxidants, serves as the foundation of this diet.

- **Other Fruits:** Pair mango with other fruits such as berries, pineapple, or kiwi for added flavor, sweetness, and variety.

- **Greek Yogurt:** Combine mango with Greek yogurt for a creamy and nutritious breakfast or snack option that's rich in protein and probiotics.

- **Nuts and Seeds:** Sprinkle chopped mango over nuts or seeds like almonds, walnuts, or chia seeds for added texture, healthy fats, and nutritional variety.

- **Whole Grains:** Serve mango alongside whole grains like quinoa, brown rice, or whole grain toast for added fiber and sustained energy.

Instructions:

1. **Mango Smoothie:** Blend mango chunks into smoothies along with other fruits, leafy greens, Greek yogurt, nut milk, and a scoop of protein powder for a tropical and refreshing beverage that's packed with vitamins, minerals, and protein.

2. **Mango Salsa:** Dice mango and combine with chopped tomatoes, onions, cilantro, jalapeno, lime juice, and a pinch of salt for a flavorful and vibrant salsa that pairs well with grilled fish or chicken.

3. **Mango Salad:** Combine sliced mango with mixed greens, avocado, red onion, toasted nuts, and a citrus vinaigrette for a refreshing and nutrient-rich salad that's perfect for summer.

4. **Mango Chia Pudding:** Mix pureed mango with chia seeds and almond milk, then let it sit in the fridge until thickened for a creamy and satisfying pudding that's rich in fiber, protein, and omega-3 fatty acids.

5. **Mango Sorbet:** Blend frozen mango chunks with a splash of coconut water or orange juice until smooth, then freeze until firm for a refreshing and healthy dessert option that's perfect for hot days.

Artichokes Diet

Definition: The artichokes diet involves incorporating artichokes as a nutritious and flavorful vegetable into meals. Artichokes are low in calories, rich in fiber, vitamins (such as vitamin C and vitamin K), minerals (such as potassium and magnesium), and antioxidants, making them a valuable addition to any diet.

Ingredients:

- **Artichokes:** The star ingredient, rich in fiber, vitamins, minerals, and antioxidants, serves as the foundation of this diet.

- **Dips:** Serve steamed or roasted artichokes with dips such as garlic aioli, lemon butter, or tahini for added flavor and indulgence.

- **Salads:** Add cooked artichoke hearts to salads along with mixed greens, tomatoes, cucumbers, olives, and feta cheese for a refreshing and nutrient-rich salad option.

- **Pasta:** Toss cooked artichoke hearts with whole grain pasta, cherry tomatoes, spinach, garlic, and olive oil for a light and flavorful pasta dish that's perfect for summer.

- **Pizza:** Top pizza dough with tomato sauce, mozzarella cheese, cooked artichoke hearts, roasted red peppers, and fresh basil for a delicious and gourmet pizza option.

Instructions:

1. **Steamed Artichokes:** Steam whole artichokes until tender, then serve with a side of melted butter or aioli for dipping for a simple and delicious appetizer or side dish option.

2. **Stuffed Artichokes:** Hollow out cooked artichokes and fill with a mixture of breadcrumbs, garlic, herbs, and Parmesan cheese, then bake until golden and crispy for a flavorful and indulgent appetizer or main dish option.

3. **Artichoke Dip:** Blend cooked artichoke hearts with Greek yogurt, garlic, lemon juice, and Parmesan cheese until smooth for a creamy and flavorful dip that's perfect for serving with crackers, bread, or vegetable sticks.

4. **Artichoke and Spinach Quiche:** Mix cooked artichoke hearts with sautéed spinach, onions, eggs, milk, and cheese, then pour into a pie crust and bake until set for a delicious and hearty brunch or dinner option.

5. **Grilled Artichokes:** Halve cooked artichokes and grill until charred and tender, then drizzle with olive oil and sprinkle with salt and pepper for a smoky and flavorful side dish or appetizer option.

THE END

www.ingramcontent.com/pod-product-compliance
Lightning Source LLC
Chambersburg PA
CBHW082338220526
45470CB00008B/2552